WHEN DO i GET MY SHOELACES BACK?

....a diary of a
psychotic breakdown

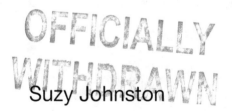
Suzy Johnston

 THE CAIRN

Published by
The Cairn,
Brincliffe,
West Dhuhill Drive,
Helensburgh G84 9AW

www.thecairn.com

A catalogue record of this book is available from the British Library.

ISBN 9780954809232

Printed by Lightning Source UK, Milton Keynes, UK

Glossary

PRN: *as required medication*

Fireboard: *board to account for which patients are present on the Ward in case of fire.*

Named Nurse: *nurse who is responsible for individual patient's care in the Ward – in my case Katy.*

Constant Observation: *nurse with you 24/7*

Friends: *Ann, Michel/Mitch, Den, Jane, Pippa, Leah*

Staff Nurses: *Katy (Named Nurse), Maxine (Student Nurse), Kim, Gary, Simon, Dawson, Clive, Keith, Lydia, Pam, Alicia, Una, Dorothy, Nikki, Alice*

Occupational Therapists: *Kathleen, Charlie*

Doctors: *Dr Smith (Consultant), Dr Fallowfield(Consultant), Dr Yaar (Senior House Officer), Dr Hamilton (Senior House Officer)*

Patients: *Miriam, Stella, Lila, Lisa*

Ward Manager: *Patrick*

Deputy Ward Manager: *Caitlin*

MDT (Multi Disciplinary Team meeting): *All sides of care e.g. doctors, nurse, occupational therapist, social worker etc meet with patient once a week to discuss care plan.*

Helpines – UK and Ireland

www.breathingspacescotland.co.uk – 0800 83 85 87 (Scotland only)

www.sane.org.uk – 0845 767 8000

www.samaritans.org.uk – 08457 90 90 90

www.aware.ie – 1890 303 302

www.nhs24.com – 0845 424 24 24

Careline – 020 8514 1177

For other countries – call your emergency health service number and ask for details of mental health support numbers/agencies.

Mental Health Websites

www.samh.org.uk
www.mind.org.uk
www.rethink.org
www.chooselife.net
www.mdf.org.uk
www.rcpsych.ac.uk
www.scottishrecovery.net
www.slam.nhs.uk
www.carers.org
www.nami.org
www.mentalhealth.org.uk
www.pendulum.org
www.seemescotland.org.uk
www.shift.org.uk
www.ru-ok.com – teens

Music and lyrics on surviving mental illness and self-harm
www.badalicemusic.com – cd/download *Walk in my Shoes.*

Foreword

It is a pleasure to be able to pen a short note of introduction to this latest book by Suzy. Written in the form of a journal, it gives the reader a 'no holds barred' and genuine account of a specific period of her life in hospital. While living through her pain, she demonstrates her courage, hope and determination to recover and tell her own story. She does this so well and gives us all a message of hope.

Breathing Space commends this touching journal to you. The subject matter is so personal and the uniqueness of the story so special. I hope that you in turn take time to look after yourself on your own journey and take the appropriate 'breathing space' you need to feel positive and well. Be uplifted and inspired!

Tony McLaren
National Coordinator, Breathing Space

To read this book is truly a privilege.

We follow a pathway of despair, distress, the highs and lows of recovery and ultimately share a very private healing. We are carried along an emotionally demanding and moving timeline, eloquently written with such feeling that pages just move by. But to read it, and absorb it, is both powerful and uplifting.

Such honesty and openness must be praised, as for many, to write (and therefore to some extent relive) would be too hard. But this journal is more than just an intensive, moving diary. It leads us to an outcome that shows how resilient we humans can be; how love, compassion and the right practical help get us through what feels like the most awful times. And that we often learn and develop as people through such adversity.

Choose Life in Argyll & Bute is proud and honoured to have played a very small part in the process that led to publication of this unique work.

Dave Bertin
Choose Life Coordinator, Argyll & Bute

ACKNOWLEDGEMENTS

I'm crap at saying thanks. And goodbyes. They make me nervous and give my legs the shakes. But this is it. Bite the bullet time. And this time it's more important than ever...

I spent approximately six and a half of the hardest months of my life in the Christie Ward during the Summer of 2008. Hard because of what was going on in my head. I nearly lost myself last year. But that wasn't allowed to happen because of a brilliant team of psychiatric staff (doctors, nurses and auxiliaries) who were there to help me, push me and drag me through the mire at just the right times. I should single them all out and shower them with plaudits but I'm afraid there isn't enough room on this page for that. My apologies. But a billion thanks anyway.

Instead, on behalf of the whole staff, I will single out two nurses, Katy and Caitlin for their unswerving care, patience, professionalism and good humour. Without them, and others, I might well have ended up on constants, on a Section or possibly even dead. I shudder at the thought. They both encouraged me to keep this diary that you might(?) be about to read. For that act alone I bless them with all the Strawberry Pencils and Dolly Mixtures in the World. Thank you.

To Dr Clarke, Dr Morrison and Dr McCrudden – thank you from the deepest, darkest recesses of my liver.

To Lomond Advocacy Service and all the staff there.

To Breathing Space and Choose Life for their ongoing support and endorsement of this book.

To Lee Knifton who has been a huge support.

To the Scottish Recovery Network and NHS Education Scotland.

Thanks to Riverdrive Studio and CGL (Oban) Ltd for designing the cover and book production assistance.

My family and friends (especially Ann and Pippa) have been UNBELIEVABLE in their help and care and as for Mitch, my now husband, he simply REFUSED to give up on me, or let me give up on myself. As with everything else in my life now I owe him everything – especially a BIG hug for giving me a future. He understood when to back off and when to step in and, as he has the condition himself, has a fantastic empathy for the emotions I was bombarded with.

Finally – to my cat, Casey, who waited so patiently with Mitch until I made the long journey home.

Thank you, thank you, thank you .....

Suzy Johnston Syrett
January 2010

This book is dedicated to my wonderful, funny, fantastic husband,

Michel

Introduction

Potato skins. I guess that's as good a place to start as any. Sometime on a Wednesday in the middle of January 2008 I was seated in a restaurant faced with a bowl of freshly cooked potato skins and a variety of dips and you know what? I couldn't STOMACH them. Even looking at them made me feel ill. So I ate nothing and tried to ignore the worried glances from my friend opposite.

By the time Tuesday came around I was feeling horrendous and somewhat confused as to why the "bug" I assumed I had wasn't shifting.

So I made an appointment to see my GP. I know my GP well and as I suffer from bipolar disorder and I'm on a variety of medications, I like to make a point of seeing her regularly. But this was different. I was in a bad way – I could hardly walk and everything I tried to eat was making me sick even drinking water, and keeping it down was difficult. I described as best I could to the doctor what I was experiencing but even that proved difficult as I was feeling so unwell and confused. She duly took some blood and told me to go home and that she'd be in touch if the lab reported anything.

Three hours later the phone rang. It was my doctor. She informed me that my liver was malfunctioning and that my LFT score (Liver Function Test) – which should be between 2 and 40 – was residing at 2300. This was not good. Even I realised that!

I spent the next six weeks being sick, losing a huge amount of weight, turning a fetching shade of yellow, having blood taken regularly, being sick, you get the picture. I was diagnosed with viral Hepatitis A and was told that it should clear up in a few weeks.

All seemed to be going according to plan and life returned to normal at the beginning of March. I could go out and about again, socialise and pretty much eat what I felt like. But then…THEN, at the beginning of April I started feeling horribly sick again and when I noticed that my pee had turned bright orange the warning bells started ringing and I headed straight back to my GP for another blood test. The news was not good. My LFT score had headed back up to 800 and this time I felt SO ILL I didn't know what to do with myself. However, apparently the doctors did and I found myself spending three weeks in a medical Ward in the Vale of Leven Hospital. But whilst I was there something happened that none of us realised would have such a HUGE effect on my health: ALL of my psychiatric medication (apart from my lithium which is metabolised in the kidneys) was stopped. Immediately. The result? I became paranoid, frightened, suicidal, depressed and had to cope with auditory and visual hallucinations all the while in a noisy and unfamiliar place. I also had to deal with an SHO telling me that "Bipolar is NOT an affective disorder but is a PERSONALITY disorder which doesn't respond to medication and it's up to you to snap out of it and pull yourself together." (It isn't!) So it was not the easiest time.

I was EXTREMELY frustrated that everybody was SO focused on my liver when I was SCREAMING inside my head for help with what was going on there. The divisions between medical wards and psychiatric wards had never been so highlighted for me as they were during those few weeks.

What you are about to read is the diary I kept during the six and a half months I spent in Christie Ward – The Vale of Leven's acute psychiatric unit – immediately following my transfer from the acute medical Ward. It is CRUCIAL to keep in mind that, for around the first two months I was on NO MEDICATION (other than lithium) and was totally reliant on nursing support and intervention. This book, I believe, gives a unique insight into psychosis as it occurs and poses questions and gives answers as to how those amazing people we call psychiatric nurses kept me alive and spared me as much suffering as was humanly possible. Keeping the diary was part of my therapy and it is my hope that by sharing it will serve as an educational tool as to how it feels to be, live and experience as a patient in a psychiatric Ward.

This was no easy journey.

So don't expect it to be an easy read.

WHEN DO i GET MY SHOELACES BACK?

Open letter to the Staff:

Is it normal when planning a suicide attempt to feel so cold, empty and detached that, apart from a residual feeling of sadness and impotence, the idea and visualisation of the act itself leave no tangible emotion in their wake?

I think I AM scared, but I seem to have, at least somewhere along this path, gained the very necessary ability to shut off 'troublesome' and interfering thoughts and feelings, focusing instead on the practical e.g. a washing line would probably be best (sorry this is grim).

You might think all this means I have no hope for life? Not true. If my medication and my liver get 'sorted' quickly then I have every chance of making it. What I _can't_ deal with, however, is all of this HORRIFICALLY, TORTUOUS _WAITING_. I don't think I am exaggerating when I say it's getting more and more difficult to find the focus and energy to keep going. And I'm just not sure that I want to anymore, I don't think I'm quitting – I'm just pretty convinced that my hand is not good enough and it's time to fold. No drama. No hysterics. Please.

Do I have a plan? Yes. But I'm not willing to share it with you. I'm not pissing about: I just need to know that IF I choose to go through with this option there will be minimum room for foul ups. I'm not brave enough to get caught and I reckon that this is a one shot opportunity.

I'm writing this because I'm REALLY hoping that you can help me out of this. I can't cope on my own right now and the Ward is the only place that I get even the slightest taste of safety. Everything feels as though it is going wrong and I am hindered like a sprinter with leg irons on as I STRUGGLE to manage without appropriate and therapeutic meds. This is SO difficult.

I appreciate that all of the Staff are trying really hard to help me but this is the HARDEST thing I have EVER done.

May

10th May

Sometimes I want to kill myself so much that the air grows thick with the urgency of it all. This is one of those times.

Katy ran me a scented bath at 2:00am (after checking, on my request, that the bathroom was safe for me) to try and help me chill out but I STILL COULDN'T SLEEP.

11th May 3:30pm

Feeling okay — handed over a dressing gown belt Mum inadvertently gave me... half think I did the right thing/half angry that I couldn't bring myself to keep it just in case..... s'pose it was a pretty safe bet — I couldn't have left Mum with that sort of guilt trip.

5:45pm

Don't want to tempt fate but I'm pretty nervous now that the end of the day is creeping into my bones. The night is unpredictable and never fun. Keeping my room door open helps.

13th May

Got my shoelaces, phone charger, headphones and belts taken away this evening when I confessed to Katy about my intentions to hang myself from the bathroom door. I think she knew I wasn't messing around. I knew I wasn't messing around.

Just let me be.

14th May

The problem about making it through a day is that there is always another one stepping up to take its place.

A bit nervous about seeing Ann today. I assured her last week that I wouldn't consider killing myself whilst I was still in hospital and that I had no fixed plans or methods in mind. However, entering the Christie Ward was like pulling my finger out of the dyke and the floodgates are so open that they are off their hinges. Things have changed.

Afternoon:

When a doctor tells you in the morning that he has found an antipsychotic that he thinks he can put you on and then??? Then in the afternoon he pisses over any shreds of hope that you might have saved up by telling you sorry! It's not going to happen.

Pinning your hopes on anything is stupid but I'm human and a tiny bit fragile right now so forgive me for not responding well to that enormous kick in the guts.

Don't do that again please.
Don't do that again.

17th May

I think too much about what I think

18th May

What I WANT to do and what I SHOULD do feel miles apart right now. What I WANT to do is kill myself and I am growing increasingly angry and frustrated at both the barriers being put in my way and the general apathy that is sucking at my veins. Aaargh!

What I SHOULD be doing is seeking out members of staff but I'm frightened and everything in my head screams "DANGER!"

My brain is toying with me:
There are times when I am convinced my room is bugged
Yes, I've started hallucinating again
Yes, I'm hearing background frequency in my head a lot of the time.

I can't figure out for certain the observation timings in the ward as it all seems a bit erratic and unpredictable (maybe this is deliberate?) so I can't put my Ward "plan" into operation 'cos I'm terrified that I get caught. That is my NIGHTMARE because I'm a BIG COWARD.

What else?......

Yes, I get shit scared of the staff particularly Kim — she's plotting to kill me — and as such I'm finding it increasingly difficult to approach ANY of them and ask for help which, I know, is self defeating at best and stupid and dangerous at worst but it's SO HARD when you are SURE that people are going to assault you if they are given even the tiniest chance. How to explain this conflict of ideas..... It's like my brain is trying to shut down every avenue of help available to me ANYWHERE and I become convinced that I am the worst type of burden, a right royal pain in the ass and that I should just pull my finger out, quit moaning and just get on with killing myself. I realise that right now

(9.15am) and in the cold (hot!) daylight that perhaps none of this is true, but I also suspect that in about 10 hours things could look very different again.

I HATE this with everything that I am which is part of the reason I want "out" of this SO MUCH but I'm trying really hard to lay the biggest guilt trip on myself and remind myself that I don't want to hurt ANYBODY ELSE. I just don't know if that will be reason enough and at the moment I doubt it.

19th May 6:00am

I'm tired. This seems to get harder every day and I'm struggling under the heavy weight of all of these bad thoughts. I know I should seek help when things get tough but it never seems quite that clear cut and easy. I'm frightened that people will start to give up on me because I'm not sure I can do this on my own.

Tried to convince Michel to stop visiting but he's having none of it. The reason for this request? The big piece of me that wants to die right now figured I might find it easier if he was kept at a distance. Thankfully there's a little bit of me that's glad he's such a stubborn git. I'm trying and trying and trying but I'm just at the beginning of this journey and I honestly don't have a clue where it will end. I don't want to think about it too much – I've never fallen into this particular tunnel so I'm a bit lost and it's easy to walk away from the light when your eyes are glued shut.

12:15pm

I think that I'm going to lose.
It seems as though I have two reasonable options here:
1. Get back on medication ASAP
2. Hang myself

20th May

I don't seem to take disappointments too well at the moment and I ricochet from them with all the unpredictability of a desperate bonus ball in a crazed pin ball machine. If I don't get to see Dr Smith today that will be a LITTLE bit tough to deal with because obviously it means SEVEN DAYS AND NIGHTS until my next chance. That pushes me to (beyond?) my limits and makes my "hanging on fingernails" peel and shred. I can smell the breath of constant observations and that whole concept is SO paranoia inducing that it is terrifying. I'm finding it hard enough to be around staff and the idea that at least one of them could be in my face ALL THE TIME scares me witless. I know it's for my safety but at what price in the longer term? Because if it happens it has to end sometime and then?

21st May

You'd think you'd notice when a large plank smacks you on the side of the head. That is what this feels like. The suicidal thoughts are immense and hit me hard and without warning, leaving me bewildered, nauseous and as freaked out as a wet cat. Of course from experience I know that they only last an hour. ONLY an hour? ONLY a lifetime, that's all.

So far I have muddled scrambled and hobbled my way through. I HAVE gone for help (against my better/worse judgement) because coping strategies do little more than tickle the surface when it is THIS BAD and I don't know what the fuck else to do. This is not ME, not anything, just a stumbling shell filled with death and unhealthy desires and, like badly fitting shoes, it cripples and leaves unwelcome bruises in its wake.

PM:

Became certain that doctors and day staff were having secret meetings about me and saying AWFUL THINGS and plotting how they were going to get rid of me. I was terrified. (And you wonder why I keep thinking about killing myself???) WHAT IF THE PILLS DON'T WORK AND THIS KEEPS HAPPENING?!!!

Oh my God.

June

9th June

Too many things make sense right now like how my lithium is a placebo (or sometimes I wonder if it might be tampered with). I don't know. But what I DO know is that my gut instinct is SCREAMING at me not to take it. So what do I do? I allow the white pills to work their way down into my nervous system and so give them licence to do what they will. How weak am I? Afterwards I don't feel at all mood stabilised just frightened, angry and upset. I don't want to be any of those things.

Using my phone right now is a complicated and wearing process. It's crap. Basically I HAVE to be in my bathroom with BOTH doors shut or else everyone else in the Ward can listen in to my calls (which sucks). I realise, or at least a tiny bit of me does that this is irrational but I can't risk not being safe, so the bathroom it is.

Someone is going to give me a kicking tonight – maybe more than one person. A vitriolic seed has been planted in my head and it's whispering louder and louder in a very convincing manner that it's most likely to be the night staff. It's a fair bet that I will be held down whilst one of them, I'm not sure who, belts me. Please understand how much I HATE feeling like this. EVERY NIGHT. I have NO control over what I think or believe at the moment and it terrifies me. I AM NOT NORMALLY LIKE THIS. REALLY.

10th June

How is it possible to feel this unhappy and still be able to force my face into some sort of smile? Things are looking up in my MDT so I should be chuffed right? But, for God's sake, NO ANTIPSYCHOTIC PRN, NO ANTISYCHOTIC PRN, NO ANTIPSYCHOTIC PRN!!! I think I am going to fucking die. PLEASE spare me that thing of saying "Hey, everything else is really good" because without the PRN I am going to have to crawl on bloody knees to make it through the night and sometimes I'm not even sure I want to try.

Things are BAD right now and I HATE IT ALL.

Paranoia/suicidal thoughts/hallucinations? Feel free to pick which one will raise it's head tonight 'cos I don't have a CLUE.

11th June 5:30am

Still unsure about things. The "things" in question being my vulnerability/potential for harm of taking lithium. I only took it yesterday because I felt pretty intimidated by Simon. If I had a strong bone in my body (apparently I don't) I would say "Sod it", not take it and just walk away. The problem is I don't know who I'm most scared of — lithium or the nurses.

Two more things. Dr Yaar was upstairs last night plotting against me with the other faceless doctors. He's in charge now that Dr Smith is away and that TERRIFIES me.

Other thoughts again during the night were that the night staff were going to assault me. The door to the ward is locked at night and there is nowhere to run to. Nowhere. Clive gave me his word that I was safe but I just couldn't trust him in my head.

I'm so many things right now — frightened, hopeless, confused, disappointed, angry and upset. I cried for the first time in AGES yesterday and I don't think that's a good sign because it indicates that I'm starting to lose my grip when I'm trying so hard to keep it together.

12th June 5:45am

The things I'm saying at night make me cringe first thing in the morning. It's no fun waking up humiliated, embarrassed and a little confused because somewhere deep inside something is still whispering to me that it's all true.

Last night? I dunno. It all got a bit complicated and I was sure there was some doctor/nurse led conspiracy against me. STILL DON'T TRUST DR YAAR BECAUSE HE'S BEHIND ALL THIS.

Also accused Lydia of "being against me" and being pissed off with me which I see now was a TERRIBLE thing to do. She's doing a great job of trying to get me to challenge my thoughts (not the easiest thing in the world). So what do I do? Figure that all the staff are having a good laugh about me behind my back.

I KNOW that this is paranoia but I am SURE that people are following me and stalking me. Great. Suicidal thoughts reared in my head last night but as if in some twisted horse race they were beaten to the post by paranoid thoughts which celebrated their victory by parading around my head all night.

14th June

I don't even want to THINK about yesterday, but then that's not really an option is it as I'm writing this diary and the fact that memories of how I felt/thought/was desperate to kill myself but too bloody, BLOODY CHICKEN to go through with it continue to circumnavigate my skull. I am so SICK of my constant failings and 'wimp outs'. WHY do I keep fighting this??? WHY? That's the question that literally makes me vomit. This is not an easy road and I have NO idea where it ends.

A secret: I have ALWAYS believed, for as long as I can remember, that I would die by killing myself. I just never figured when. I realise that this sounds horrendously morbid. Sorry. It just feels awfully close at the moment, that's all.

My brain was like a bike with a broken chain yesterday, constantly slipping out of gear and coming to a jarring halt over and over again. I actually felt as though I was slightly concussed – no headache just a 'stunned' feeling and I was finding it really hard just to generally function.

Last night was the LONGEST, TOUGHEST night of my life. My plans are not abstract but live things that prod and taunt me CONTINUOUSLY. I slept for about 2 hrs and the rest of the time was "Should I? Shouldn't I?" I didn't go for help. The paranoia made sure of that.

My Named Nurse, Katy, asked me why I had come up and approached her twice earlier in the evening about trivial stuff? BECAUSE I GET SCARED! It's hard just to come out with the big bad things so sometimes I need to build up.

15th June

There was another secret doctors' meeting about me last night upstairs and whilst I realise I'm not that fascinating or important I was still SURE that EVERY phone call, fax or email in the office was about me and passing information about my case and notes.

The thing that's worrying me most at the moment though is that the staff have given up on me and are, at best, discarding and, at worst, disbelieving EVERYTHING I have to say. THE PILLS AREN'T WORKING and all I have left is the staff. I can't do this on my own. I CAN'T DO THIS ON MY OWN! _REALLY_.

16th June

PARANIOA SUCKS AND I FUCKING HATE THE WAY IT MANGLES MY BRAIN. I think weird shit about people, about meetings, about bloody FOLDERS for God's sake.

So. BIG chat with Dr Fallowfield and the end up is that he has encouraged me to go ahead with my complaints about Dr Yaar and that Dr Yaar will no longer be my SHO. This is not a character assassination. Sure, the guy scares the living SHIT out of me but I strongly feel that NO ONE should go through the admissions process I did ie in the very public presence of 5 other people in another Ward. Dr Fallowfield will now take my MDTs until Dr Smith returns.

Brain went 'phut' again and sllllllooooooooowwwwwyyyyy ground to a halt allowing suicidal thoughts to run riot for around 1½ hrs. Tried to speak to Pam but I was crap, crap, crap and felt so zoned out that I could barely keep my eyes open.

Maybe I am the most selfish, negative person in the World. Maybe I am. The evidence? 1. I'm not there for Mitch when he needs me. I'm pushing him away and he's in a bad state at the moment. I can't help it. I have other even more pressing things on my mind that for both our sakes I need to be ever vigilant and focused about. Why? Because that's ALL I can do. Yes most of the time I AM winning but "most" isn't close to being "always" and when I'm feeling okay that worries me. When I'm not feeling okay it's a whole different story and it DOESN'T WORRY ME AT ALL.

Maybe it's a cop out but when someone BELTS you over the head/flicks a switch in your brain and you start being preoccupied with really bad stuff then it's hard to turn that whole mindset into something else. I feel a radio tuned into a BAD programme and the dial's stuck. I'm in a whole, new, monster of a "tunnel" and I don't have a clue what I'm doing nevermind THINKING half the time.

But you've probably heard all of this before.
Boring, isn't it?

pm:
Right now I'm scared to write down what I'm thinking and how I feel. I CAN'T get a member of staff so this is down to me. Enough. ENOUGH! ENOUGH!!!

CAN'T SEEM TO GET THE THOUGHTS TO BACK THE HELL OFF!!!

Feeling LOADS better. Should've gone and got Lydia at the time. Duh. I just get in the way of myself sometimes and that can/could be dangerous. But right now. I'm okay. So I'll try and focus on that for now.

17th June

Started out well with a good chat with Dorothy and felt in good spirits until a short while later when KERPOW paranoid thoughts and suicidal thoughts came rocking into my skull and decided to hold a very loud and destructive party and wreck the inside of my head.

Note to self: apparently my HAT is a dead giveaway that I am feeling crap. The REASON I wear it is that I feel that it helps contain the thoughts and if it helps I'm going to continue doing it. Just wish it wasn't such a beacon though!

Felt pretty horrible for about 1½ hrs all the same symptoms as usual except I thought Lydia was saying awful things about me JUST out of earshot and that Dr Yaar was having a right laugh at me — in fact ALL I could see for a while when I closed my eyes — even blinked — was his face contorted in hysterical laughter. Not pleasant. Spoke to Dorothy about this which helped a bit.

18th June

And so the thoughts begin. I can feel suicidal impulses crawling around my brain like deranged spiders. PLEASE GO AWAY. Without an antipsychotic PRN I feel like a beginner swimmer without armbands. I'm fucking drowning here — the psychotic thoughts just get magnified and it totally sucks.

FIVE hours of continuous, RELENTLESS suicidal thoughts tears at your soul. I found that I couldn't walk straight, felt stunned, had a hard job focusing and keeping my eyes open. What the Hell is going on with me?

I am pre-empting NOTHING.

This WILL happen again and it scares the shit out of me.

Still feeling really depressed despite Katy telling me a funny story that made me smile despite myself.

19th June

Pretty GREAT morning and slept until 6.00am. Felt good and relaxed until 11ish when suicidal thoughts began to appear like unwelcome mould on a birthday cake. I. Should. Know. Better. As ever it was only a matter of minutes before EVERYTHING escalated and a large and very solid baseball bat came crashing down on my head. If this was a cartoon, fragments of bone, blood and brain would spatter everywhere but in this reality there is nothing tangible to see. But boy, do I FEEL it! My head is stuffed to bursting with thoughts of death and the accompanying visualisations are HORRIFIC. I get very, VERY scared until... until it reaches the dangerous phase where all fear melts and I feel no consideration for anyone or anything.

Still felt shitty when Mitch came to visit and got too edgy for a walk beyond the car park. And then? Then it passed. How or why I don't know. But from 3.00pm up until now 7.00pm all is well.

20th June

I think even my memory has decided it doesn't want to be a part of this anymore. Psychosis? Self protection? Mortification??? I don't know. What I DO know is that when my head caved in last night ALL I could think of was finding some way out of that very, VERY solid and locked front door and hanging myself. Simon wasn't up for it so we had a big chat instead. I threw up afterwards but at least I got a good night's sleep which was cool.

1:15pm

GOOD morning but slightly suspicious of Alicia as she gave me a weird look when she told me there was nothing mentioned in my file about last night. Nope. Don't believe her. Feel like the whole World's against me today and I SWEAR TO GOD that Dr Yaar is stalking me — EVERY time I walk down the office corridor he appears. Shit.

3:20pm

VERY suspicious of Alicia and when I confronted her she went to show me my notes. But..............what if there are TWO copies though — one for patients to be shown and a totally different version for nurses and doctors??? My version looked fine but I'm still nervous about the other one which I want shredded. Yes, I'm sure that there is a conspiracy against me involving the staff and medics. More secret meetings, photocopies, faxes and emails against me and about me...

Evening: WHY IS THIS HAPPENING? Paranoid as FUCK again tonight. Started when I thought Una acted a little strange when I said "hello" to her and quickly EXPLODED into certainty that she was planning to batter me when I was asleep. Nice. Terrified, I confronted her and she denied everything. Didn't believe her. So she sent me to listen to my MP3 player. I did this for about 15 mins when the thought "She wants me out of her hair so she can plan to hurt me!" SLAMMED into my brain. I charged into the office and she denied this too and as apparently I looked knackered, sent me to bed.

21st June

Got up and immediately apologised to Una. I can be SUCH a SHIT at times and I'm sorry for that.

12:00pm

The suicidal thoughts that have in turn, been lurking, pestering and, finally, overwhelming this morning are on the wane (thank God). There was a trigger this time – a dangerous looking idle hairdryer all on it's lonesome in the bathroom. If you had turned the volume up you would have heard it SCREAMING HANG YOURSELF, HANG YOURSELF, HANG YOURSELF. Got Patrick who removed it. Unfortunately he couldn't remove the domino effect it had started in my head.

6:00pm

I AM SO SICK OF ALL OF THIS!!!!!!!!!!!!! When the thoughts grow in my head like deranged acorns on speed all: I. Can. THINK. ABOUT. IS . HANGING. MYSELF.
And it's knackering.
And it's scary.
And I feel out of control.

And I can't see a way out.
And I FUCKING HATE it.

7:00pm

Why the Hell is there a nurse here spying on me? I don't know her and I don't trust her. Why was she doing the Fire Board? Plus she looks at me funny and generally scares me. A lot.

22nd June

The REALLY crap thing about last night's paranoia is how ORDINARY AND EXPECTED It's all become. Still scares the shit out of me though. Completely. I'm SO sick of having to face down my fears (literally at times). SO SICK OF IT. Last night I copped out and offloaded on Lydia. Twice. And it was getting worse — I started thinking Caitlin wasn't really a nurse but had been sent to spy on me and was acting well weird — taking notes and stuff. All I wanted to do was go to sleep and get the hell away from my head. But it's never that easy is it?

11:45am

I HATE myself and I can feel the hate rotting like fungus from within. I know all too well where this is going. Don't let it last too long. I'm tired today.

4:30pm

At last. Some respite. I'm not dead anymore and, for just now, I can feel the warmth of taking a breath, of seeing clearly, of being able to think rationally. No more analysing and writing — I'm just going to enjoy this for a bit.

8:50pm

NO! I can feel the beginnings of 'interference' in my head. HOW DO I STOP IT???

23rd June 5:20am

I felt awful last night plagued by thoughts that my phonecalls were being broadcasted and that EVERYONE in here was talking about me. Plus I couldn't stop seeing myself hanging and actually FEELING a noose around my neck.

Spoke to Lydia about suicidal thoughts versus getting better. Lydia thinks I'm impatient. She's wrong. This is one patient patient when I need to be. The reason I get up at 5:00am? Because between 5-9am I can be fairly sure that I'll be feeling okay AND I WANT AS MUCH OF THAT AS POSSIBLE. Maybe I'm stupid. Maybe I'm greedy? But normality is SO important and I won't, CAN'T waste it. I need to savour it as much as possible.

12:30pm

I've decided that I'm NOT going to try to leg it. That would entail 2 things: 1. People looking for me; 2. Everything rushed.

Neither appeals. I don't know if I can be saved. I just don't know. I accept the final responsibility is mine — the staff can only do so much and the medication isn't fucking working. I also accept that hanging myself will be absolutely horrendous but at least it's finite whereas the chaos in my head is AGONISING in its endlessness.

I don't know what's going to happen.

5:50pm

Trying but can't seem to shake these thoughts that coat my body and brain like unwelcome ghosts. Feeling better than earlier but the thoughts are STILL THERE. Relentless and mocking. Dull and terrifying. And under it all? A plan that SCREAMS my name. Hard to ignore, impossible to erase. I'm doing ALL THE RIGHT THINGS and still the idea of doing the wrong things has times of HUGE appeal. WHY??? Taking my medication is like swimming underwater – I have to come up for air sometime and it is then, tired and vulnerable, that the eager horror thoughts pounce again and mentally nail gun me to a very solid wall.

Y'know what? I'm starting not to care much anymore and I'm very, VERY tired of all of this.

Is Dorothy saying horrible things about me? Are the staff secretly wanting me to come to harm? I'm just NOT SURE and it's doing my HEAD in. I don't seem to have any internal barometer to tell me what's real and what's not. So I am suspicious of EVERYTHING and it burns holes in my brain.

24th June 5:15am

Those suicidal thoughts just wouldn't shift last night, and they had the temerity to invade my sleep – hence up at 4:00am today. No paranoia though. Got a bit wary of Kim at one point but managed to 'nip it in the bud' by checking if she was cool with me or if there was a problem. However, I am sure the staff are talking about me RIGHT NOW so I have got up to check them out. Suicidal thoughts? I can laugh, chat, banter but when you strip all of that away you can't get away from the broken "kill yourself" record that endlessly grinds round and round SHRIEKING through its weary needle. So. I need to keep focused and use the distraction techniques that the nurses are helping me with. It's just SO HARD. First thing in the morning is when things are at their best but I get tired later and distracted and that's when things become a big problem. NOTHING gets a look in at those times and it alarms me how lacking in fear I am becoming.

MDT with Dr Fallowfield today. Antipsychotic PRN?

2:45pm
How emotions change. Three hours ago I was ecstatic to be given an antipsychotic PRN. Now three hours later? IT DOESN'T FUCKING WORK. At least not so that I'd notice. Empty promises SUCK. I'm angry, bitter, frustrated and upset. Super. Demons are playing in my head again and their games will only get faster paced and more demented. This I have learned every day since April 1st when this all started. Some fool me.

5:30pm
I HATE MY LIVER. My brain is screaming for therapeutic medication but my fucking liver ALWAYS has to put up its hand and say "Excuse me? No!" All I want is something that I can take when I feel bad that will, partially at least, alleviate the daymare/nightmare in my head. That's all. WHY is this so DIFFICULT? 'Angry' only scratches at the surface. I'm depending on this. Get that? DEPENDING.

8:00pm

My plan is firmly locked in my brain and though I feel fine right now I can still all too clearly hear its squeaky cogs turning. Sometimes I get a break and, like an obliging neighbour, the volume is turned down. But it's ALWAYS there and it's wearing me down. The paranoia thinks this is HYSTERicaL AND gleefully takes any opportunity to join the party. I NEED this to STOP. NOW. LATER is just too dangerous.

It took 5½ hours to get through that last episode. Yes, I got through it but my pulse of 118bpm demonstrates the physical aspect never mind the mental side of things. I've spoken about this SO much that I won't bore you by repeating it. Mental torment is such a regular feature in day/nighttime right now that I am totally resigned to it. I think I am beginning to give in, which part of me knows is weak and wrong but another part really just wants this to be finished. What it is coming down to is a race between medication and support and hanging myself. I can't even begin to figure out the odds but at the moment my faith and belief in myself and my future is shaky at best.

If I could I would cry and NEVER stop.

ELEMENTAL by Me

The darkness spreads inside me
And I'm scared and lost within
I'm not afraid to say I'm losing
And that my soul is wearing thin

I'll do my best not to complain
But something is amiss
I know my thoughts aren't normal
What made me come to this?

And in the dark all I can hear's my breath
Don't you know that I'm scared to death?
I can't fly away like I used to do
Delusions broke off my wings and left me bleeding too...too...too

And if I have the option
I know I have a choice
Don't try to tell me I can't make it
I HAVE to find my voice

Elemental
Elemental

25th June 5:25am

I think I might be sick. This morning I feel as though my insides have been coated with lead and my heart petrified and turned to stone. My brain won't let me sleep too long — just enough time to recover from the ragged, scrambled, suicidal mess that was my World last night but not long enough — NOT LONG ENOUGH to heal and let me forget the way it torments. I feel despondent today and I'm trying hard to get a sense of myself in all this but IT'S NOT WORKING. Where the Hell have I gone? God, I LOATHE this and the PRN isn't helping. I want to STOP TIME. Yes, this all negative but I need to spew my guts and vitriol all over this page or else it stays inside. And it BURNS.

10:45am

Here it comes again. Here it comes again. Here it comes again. I know only too well that I have around 30 mins before my brain dies and is replaced by a clanking engine of self hate and suicidal thoughts. AND I CAN'T STOP IT... AND IT TERRIFIES ME!!! A PRN that DOESN'T DO ANYTHING and coping strategies that are as resilient as shreds of tissue paper in a rainstorm are ALL I HAVE if I am to do this alone. But I can't. So I bother and bother and BOTHER the staff (whom I am jealous of for their clear heads, lack of psychosis and easy confidence). This is SHIT.

6:10pm

Spent from 1:30pm onwards accusing Caitlin of having it in for me, sending my notes (and photocopying them) to 'doctors' who are planning to harm/kill me. Great. Feel better now (Did the PRN help?) Worried that I've damaged my good relationship with Caitlin. It all started with what I perceived as a weird look from her then BAM it all kicked off. I tried to nip it in the bud by confronting her but that just made things worse. HOW DO I STOP THIS SICKO ROLLERCOASTER? And how do I get off???

I HATE THIS SO MUCH

8:00pm

I fell pretty fed up at the minute, as though I've let myself down and that I SHOULD be able to control the paranoia regardless of how 'real' it seems.

Anyway, it's early and I'm already scared of later.

26th June 5:20am

The staff must be SICK of me. I'M sick of me. Last night was GREAT until around 10:00pm ish when bad thoughts and paranoia hounded me like a swarm of angry and "We're out to sting" wasps. And guess what folks? I wake up feeling more or less the same. Fanfuckingtastic. I'm tempted to try and get Kim or Una to open the door but I'm not THAT stupid and DON'T want to see a psychiatrist right now. The consequences are WAY too uncertain and threatening. Anyway, Kim or Una would speak to the psych before I could and it would be a fait accompli. I don't stand a chance and being sectioned or transferred aren't on my Christmas wish list.

Got to try those distraction techniques 'cos the PRNs just aren't working so distraction techniques are all I have to try and beat this (mocking laughter pervades.) I'm going to sit in reception and listen to my MP3 player. I'll take it from there.

Felt as suicidal as a lemming through the night and got up to query Kim about my rights as an informal patient. I wanted out in both senses of the word SO BADLY. She warned me off and it didn't take a genius to realise that I would be going nowhere. That door was staying locked.

Slept from 1am — 3:45am

8:45am

Feeling much better and kind of like my old self! All right!

10:00am

A little bit edgy and I can smell darkness and see shapes on the not too distant horizon. I'm panicking a bit if I'm honest.

2:05pm

Wow, I felt like SHIT earlier. The smash — yer — head — in cricket bat hit home HARD at around 10:30am and I SIMPLY COULDN'T THINK of anything other than HANGING MYSELF. There was no room for distraction, no room for conversation and no room for ME so I bailed out of the group I was in and retreated, licking my seeping, aching wounds, to under my duvet with my MP3 player blaring God knows what. I kind of felt that I fell into some kind of mental 'coma' for sometime as I definitely didn't sleep — there was too much noise in my head for that — but I lost about an hour that I can't account for. This is CRAP and I have NO IDEA what to do about it.

Had a good lunch hour with Pippa — felt a little nervous but the tearoom was fairly empty so I was okay. Gave Pippa the "15" version of events eg. admitted and described paranoia but didn't talk about suicidal thoughts. Did the same with Jane on the phone. Can't bring myself to tell my friends the truth which in some ways is a terrible thing but in others easier for everyone.

27th June 6:35am

Wanted to kill myself again last night. Wanted Pam or Lydia to let me out of the front door. Wanted both SO BAD I could taste them. Neither happened. Distractional technique of a freezing cold shower helps dissipate some of the residual anger that I was harbouring. Note to self: must try harder with distraction if I'm going to survive this.

10:00am

Feel fine mentally and I've had a good morning so far.

12:40pm

Reasons that things might be good:
1. Marrying Mitch
2. Moving in with Mitch
3. New book to be published
4. Sessional job still waiting?
5. Recording new band music?
6. Back to normal health wise

5:30pm

This is seemingly ENDLESS today. I'm AFRAID (which in some ways is a good thing), and I'm having trouble even wanting to be in the same room as myself at the moment. I feel like too many bad things to mention. I can't be bothered AND I'm so melodramatic. If I feel dead already what's the point in my external existence? I can't believe this is still happening. I can't believe in my future. I can't believe in myself. I can't believe.

I KNOW I'm being negative but if I wrote about how full of hope and positivity I am right now I'd be a liar as well as all my other failings. So humour me. At least for a short while.

I need to get all of this stuff out of my head and onto paper where I stand a greater chance of being able to rationalize things. That's the idea anyway. Who knows if it'll work?

9:35pm

I have been feeling it now like bad rain in the air for the past 20 mins. EVERYTHING becomes that much harder: making jokes, making SENSE, responding to others, being around people. And the fear is rising and tangible — but it's like liquid tar and slips through my fingers when I try to push it away.

I don't know what tonight will bring but I DO KNOW that I'm scared already and it's early yet. A big part of me wants to shut everyone out tonight – I've socialised, chatted, had a bit of banter, ENOUGH!!! I have things to figure out and I can do without the distraction. It is SO tempting to do this and let things follow their natural course. But if 'consequences' are to be avoided (although I can already feel the anger BURNING) I. MUST. TALK. TO. THE. STAFF. (Please feel free to raise a hand if you can spot the manipulated patient) I WANT OUT! THIS ISN'T FAIR!!! AAAARRRGGGHHH!!!!!

I may BE safe right now but I DON'T FEEL it. Maybe I'll be okay.

'Maybe' is a dangerous word and offers WAY too many options. I'm tied up in the boot of a car with no driver and the accelerator nailed to the floor. SHIT. PRN'S worked a treat hasn't it? What a joke. And it's not even slightly funny.

28th June 6:25am

Two new staff on the Ward and I'm already feeling nervous and suspicious of them. GODDAMNIT – one of them, Nikki, will be supervising me today. Fuck this. I feel so scared I could vomit. This is not good.

11:00am

Went for a walk with Nikki. She's all right. I still feel a bit freaked out but not as bad which is a good thing. She didn't leap in with any hard questions which I appreciated. I HOPE I can trust her 'cos right now I'm feeling like people are spying on me.

1:15pm

Feeling a little worse – suicidal thoughts mainly and a touch of paranoia. I HATE THIS SO MUCH. Nikki came and supervised me drying my hair which wasn't good. Sometimes I just want there to be NOTHING anymore.

2:20pm

My head is starting to implode and all I can do is watch the show. I WILL persevere with my distraction techniques e.g. listening to music, writing THIS but they are as ineffectual at the moment as juggling sand. I'm nervous about going for help and even handing a box of chocolates to Kim was a NIGHTMARE – felt like puking and crying but did neither because I don't have the 'balls'. Just want to be let out for 15minutes on my own.

At least, the thoughts, which are starting to dominate, do.

4:05pm

Feeling a little more connected and in control. Didn't sleep though 'cos I'm VERY scared of the thoughts returning (this is NOT pre-empting anything just accepting how things work right now). Talking with Nikki was mostly good/ a little bad. The 'good' stuff was that she met the thoughts head on and with no fear – both things I was in no shape to do on my own – which gave me confidence that MAYBE she might be able to help me through this. And, importantly, her suggestions WORKED (at least to some extent) which is pretty fucking GREAT in my book.

The 'bad' was that the paranoia kicked off again. I was pretty damn scared talking to her the first time round and I'm still nervous about constants and about who has access to my notes and diaries. So I'm a bit tired and paranoid but I feel in a better place to deal with all of this. At least for now.

5:30pm

The thoughts still grate like a bad song being played both too loudly and at the wrong speed inside my brain, BUT I feel 80% back to normal. Of course I know it will return (and that TERRIFIES me.) I just need to try and make sure it goes away.

...Even if that means LIVING in a FREEZING SHOWER.

29th June 6:05am

I am sure Dawson hates me and I have no doubt I was a right royal pain in the ass last night. I always am. Once again I'm a bit sketchy about what I actually said last night which worries me. Saying "I hate this" sounds SO weak and doesn't BEGIN to touch the angst, vitriol and self loathing that I have in me right now. I want to SCREAM and CRY and YELL but that's just not socially acceptable is it? FUCK THIS — ALL OF IT.

Also worried that ALL the staff dislike me INTENSLY. Can't gauge if this is real or paranoia — my internal mechanism for doing that appears to be broken so I have no ability to judge what is or isn't real. Great.

Moan alert: I am tired of trying, tired of fighting, tired of being hopeful and tired of being tired. I want this to be over, ONE WAY OR ANOTHER. THAT'S ALL.

9:00am
Poetry Corner (oh joy)

> *The Rain*
> *The rain pours down*
> *It beats on me*
> *But there's no water*
> *So no one notices*
> *That*
> *I'm*
> *Soaked*
> *Through.*

11:00am
The thoughts tighten round my brain like some razor wielding vice and it feels as though my head is slowly filling with blood, pus and DANGER. Thoughts of death and "actually this is starting to make sense" flood in and scare me witless. I can barely keep my eyes open — the shutters are very literally coming down. FUCK THIS. FUCK THIS. It's damaging, foul, painful and ultimately dangerous. I can't seem to stop it. And then? Then I go numb and start to WANT it. ALL of it.

11:35am
The staff are up to something. I think they are plotting against me — either to do SOMETHING to me or put me on constants.

12:30pm
My LFTs (Liver Function Tests) have tested my patience long and hard but Dr Hamilton informs me that they are now normal

so PLEASE can that mean an antipsychotic PRN that actually DOES SOMETHING. **PLEASE!!!**

2:50pm

The day I give up my planned 'hanging location' will be a day for celebration (IF it happens) but TODAY is NOT that day so DON'T PUSH ME PLEASE.

STILL PARANOID but dealing with it a bit better — issues are spiralling less and things feel a little more contained. Glad Nikki understood (I think) about how the RELENTLESS focus on my liver is pissing me off. MASSIVELY. I feel it's time to change view point and priority. It is my MENTAL HEALTH that is in crisis NOT my liver and my head NEEDS to get sorted SOON.

5:10pm
AND TONIGHT IS STILL TO COME...

7:00pm

Good visit from Mitch — he was in good spirits and it was easy to roll off jokes whilst not giving too much away and keeping tabs on the inside of my head.

8:00pm

I'm losing ME and this strange freak show is all too eager step in and take over and over and over, until nothing of what is recognisable as Suzy J remains. This is probably because I am CRAP and lousy at distracting myself. The problem is two fold 1. It's just too BIG to manage and 2. I GET SCARED. I'm human and I can't be perfect (which is pretty damn obvious).

This whole situation scares the living shit out of me and that is why I am sitting here writing this at around 8:00pm because I HAVE GOT to find a way of breaking this 'cos it's getting harder to deal with every night.

9:10pm

Since 7:30pm I have read, played my guitar (twice), listened to music, eaten crisps and dip, stretched, had two REALLY COLD showers and even watched football. So why is it that the thought of leaving the Ward and hanging myself is becoming more and more dominant as the evening progresses? SHIT. If I'm honest I'll say two things 1. The distractions ARE helping me keep a handle on things. 2. It IS STILL getting worse and I can't seem to STOP it. It feels like my brain is melting and I'm trying to hold it together but it's just running through my fingers. All that's left are these AWFUL thoughts. AND GOD ARE THEY AWFUL. Something is growing in my head and I don't like it.

I want to leave. I want out. I want no psychiatrists. I DON'T want to be Sectioned. That's what I'm trying to focus on. I DON'T want constants.

I HAVE TO BELIEVE I HAVE SO MUCH TO LIVE FOR OR ELSE. I HAVE TO BELIEVE IN SOME SENSE OF ME. I CAN DO THIS. I WANT THIS TO STOP.

30th June 6:30am

Don't want to leave. Christie is the ONLY place where I feel safe right now. I was sitting freaking out and hallucinating in reception up until around 2:00am last night when Katy came and took me up to the far end of the 'quiet corridor', pointed out of the window and whispered "Look." It took my eyes a short while to adjust but when they had I saw a small hedgehog eating a Dorito. "That's Hector" said Katy "He's partial to crisps." The whole episode had served me well and provided some much needed distraction that caused me to stop thinking about all of the crap that usually spins around in my head.

1:05pm

Nearly started crying when speaking to Kim which was weird. We were talking about signs that would tell me I was getting better. I said "Reading a whole book" but really that's crap. Gaining more of a sense of myself rather than feeling as though I'm thrashing around in the North Sea with no life jacket or hope of rescue would be good. I only feel fleeting glimpses of ME at the moment and to get them to last longer would be great.

2:46pm

I seem to be locked in to suicidal thoughts at the moment. It's like holding my breath – I can only get away from them for so long and then they reassert themselves. I DON'T KNOW WHY this is happening. Plus I felt paranoid about the staff and some of the patients – I believe they all know that Caitlin has raised the idea of sectioning me and that it is going to be discussed at tomorrow's MDT. Feel that because of this I can't really approach anyone for help. Kind of feel that my hands are tied behind my back right now. Got to make it through tomorrow's MDT and not be scared. It's my one chance. But I don't know what the staff will say...

I DON'T WANT to be sectioned but I'm REALLY worried about tonight. What if it all kicks off again and I ask to leave? When it's like that I'm in a WHOLE different headspace and the desire to hang myself is SO STRONG. It's like I have a TERRIBLE itch and I'm not aloud to scratch it so I've just got to sit and DEAL with it. And you wonder why I retch? And why I'm tired all the time. I'm exhausted from fighting the thoughts and constantly having to distract myself. Right, I'm off for a shower, hopefully that'll help.

9:40pm

The shower DIDN'T help and I felt like my brain was a mouldy raw egg sloshing around inside my head. Yes, I wanted to kill myself but, no, I didn't ask to leave the Ward. Which was good.

STRESSED TO BITS about MDT but chat with Lydia helped and I feel reassured that I have a good and viable plan should it be necessary. Thoughts of hanging are already beginning to fizz round my brain like I've OD'd on Cremola Foam. Right now it's ok — I can hack it. And MAYBE they'll go away on their own? Please?

July

1st July 6:01am

Last night was better. Yes, I wanted to leave and hang myself SO BAD that my chest hurt but, thank God, there was no drama, no calling doctors, no threats of section. Lydia just talked and listened to me and I think I realised that I couldn't go.

I NEED to ask to leave 'cos it's all I can think of along with hanging myself and I need to see if I have the opportunity to fulfil that compulsion. I ACHE about it. But I don't want to get detained so I find myself in the shitty position of not being able to leave (the door is locked and the staff won't let me out until I am assessed by a doctor) and knowing full well that if I'm honest — which I would HAVE to be — with the SHO I'd get Sectioned. Unfortunately all this serves to PISS ME OFF and I know all that anger is bad for me. At the time it feels as though I can't win. Right now, I realise that OF COURSE I win — I'm still here, but I know that later today I will feel the opposite again. That's just how things are right now. Plus I'm so tired ALL THE TIME 'cos of bad sleep but mostly because challenging these thoughts constantly is bloody exhausting. Fear is not an easy emotion to deal with or contain.

8:45am

To say I am worried about this MDT is like saying the Titanic 'nudged' an iceberg. I don't know why I am making jokes because I am really crapping it right now and have NO IDEA as to how

41

this will turn out. The Chinese say "May you live in interesting times." Sounds like a curse to me right now. PLEASE DON'T SECTION ME!

At least the MDT is with Dr Fallowfield and Katy both of whom I believe in and can talk to. When I next write in this diary I guess I'll have a better idea of what my immediate future holds. God, time is slow today.

1:15pm

FUCKINGWICKED MDT! I DIDN'T GET SECTIONED!!! ALL RIGHT! In fact the 'S' word wasn't even mentioned which was fine by me. Instead I get a PRN that SHOULD (fingers and toes crossed) work. Which is pretty damn cool. PLEASE PLEASE PLEASE WORK... I'm pretty fucking desperate here.

3:45pm

Feel like SHIT. It's hard to write.

9:50pm

Earlier was horrible — usual paranoid and suicidal thoughts with lots of visualisation. Didn't peak though so maybe new PRN is helping? I hope so. Can feel the bad thoughts stretching themselves awake from their slumber in the back recesses of my head. SHIT. Maybe PRN will help?

10:00pm

Starting to feel pretty rough.

2nd July 8:10am

Good news and bad news — bad news — HORRIBLE night for all the usual reasons: wanted to leave and hang myself, PRN made no impact but I'm not giving up on it — early days. Also think I got a bit paranoid last night as I was SURE I kept hearing people laughing about me in the Quiet Room. Pam was great and kept me from getting totally freaked out. Took a PRN later which didn't really make a difference but (good news) I SLEPT LIKE A HORSE! 11:30pm — 7:15am. AMAZING!

Feel fine this morning, can still sense thoughts rumbling away in the periphery but I can handle them at the moment quite easily so I'M OKAY.

5:05pm

Knackered. Suicidal thoughts are SO real, dominant and prevalent that I can almost touch them. Fuck this shit. Tried sleeping but woke up feeling the same. It's as though they are waiting for me and taunting me during my sleep. Kept on the move as much as much as possible as walking distracts and sitting/lying in the one place brings more focus and clarity to the thoughts. But I can't always do that as sometimes I just get TOO TIRED, so I zone out and lose touch with what's going on around me — kind of like shutting down for a bit.

My subconscious ravine had something different hidden in its depth today. I heard Ollie's voice on my MP3 player. He wasn't singing but speaking the lyrics of the song I was listening to. It lasted about 30 seconds and only stopped when panic made me turn it off and hand it in to the office to get away from it. Kind of scared of it now.

43

7:32pm

NO VISUAL HALLUCINATIONS FOR TWO WEEKS! Either the medication is helping, or, as they generally come in clusters, they've eased off of their own accord. Whatever, I don't care!

10:10pm

Starting to feel crap and pretty edgy. Panicking at what might happen later. Paranoia is starting to make fleeting appearances in my brain tearing my neurons apart as it does so. I feel damaged. Come on PRN! I heard my name being spoken in the smoke room and I KNOW they're talking about me...

3rd July 6:05am

I think the PRN is helping! My suicidal thoughts yesterday were still fucking hellish and intense but there was 'space' between them and they weren't as prevalent as they normally are. The whole episode lasted around five hours which was crap but even so I'm feeling tentatively hopeful.

Last night was really good until 9:30pm. I used all my distraction techniques (plus some new ones) — ordering in a take away, listening to music, taking a FREEZING shower, phoning one of my friends and even playing my new song (in an out of tune sort of way) to Pam. But, as Canute learned, there is no holding back some things and after 9:30pm everything got a bit, then TOTALLY, shit. Once again I wanted to leave and hang myself, was frightened of using my mobile and was sure that I was being discussed in the smoke room. I felt pretty wretched and took a PRN which helped.

3:27pm

The thing that began tapping inside my brain about half an hour ago is now methodically and deliberately scraping its broken and bloody fingernails down the inside of my skull. I COULD SCREAM. The thoughts are awake and I can feel them gearing up for action. Shit. I know where this will lead and it's to a place where distraction techniques are mocked. But I WILL TRY so I'll stop writing now and take a cold shower to try and shock the thoughts out of my system.

4:30pm

Feel like shit. Want to go for a walk ON MY OWN.

5:10pm

PRN

6:30pm

FEEL ABSOLUTELY FINE! I'm a bit knackered but my head feels as though a fresh, cooling breeze has blown through it and swept ALL of the bad thoughts away. I can finally relax and breathe again...

9:10pm

This is GREAT – I feel okay and it's LASTING. Maybe tonight will be my first clear night without any psychosis? (Please?) Now THAT would be very cool.

9:45pm

Feelings of black edginess begin to creep, no, POUR in around me like I'm a bird trapped in an oil slick. I WILL FIGHT THIS OFF.

4th July 7:05pm

Okay. So last night was shit in all the usual ways BUT the thoughts didn't remain as persistent and LOUD as they have previously. NO PARANOID THOUGHTS, which was pretty damn cool. I really feel as though both of my anti psychotics are working together although, to be honest, I'm not all that chuffed on being on a combination of two of them. I feel as though this whole medication regime is a bit of a "puncture repair kit" when really I need a whole new tyre ie. ONE effective anti psychotic – whatever that may be. I KNOW this makes me sound ungrateful and impatient but I feel as though my 'baseline' medication should be working to such an extent that I don't NEED a PRN. That's my hope anyway.

10:45am

Being positive and progressive are my only options if I'm going to make it out of here breathing. I have to TRY if only to give myself a chance. This is not some computer game where you get three lives and then re – start when you mess up. I have ONE life and if I fuck up it's 'game over'. Permanently. So today's tasks are: 1. Go out for first 5 minute walk ON MY OWN (under Caitlin's watchful eye...). 2. Go out with Pippa this afternoon and relax and enjoy myself. 3. No more phonecalls locked in the bathroom.

If I can manage these great, but I'm NOT going to give myself a hard time if I can't – there is already WAY too much negativity flowing through these veins of mine. I can't afford to add to it.

Five minute walk was fine barring one 10 second compulsion to run like Hell. But I managed, which was good.

2:05pm

Shit. Thought I had a handle on things but here it comes again. Can't write it down: that would only make thoughts more real. HELP.

4:05pm

Bad thoughts and paranoia lasted until 3pm. Didn't take PRN but used the very pleasant and most welcome distraction of walking Pippa's dogs with her in Balloch Country Park. A bit paranoid again but I'm dealing with it, so far.

8:30pm

I HATE myself. Too many ghosts flying around my head right now. I. CAN'T. THINK. If this was a game (and, believe me, it SO, SO, ISN'T) I would be losing because in the last 20 minutes the viciousness and fucking AGONY that are the contents of my brain have escalated. I WANT, NO, **I NEED** THIS TO STOP. And I consider killing myself by hanging a viable and reasonable option. I don't feel like I exist anyway so why not? My insides are rotten and coated with lead. Noise of any sort makes me wince and feel as though my head is about to EXPLODE!!!

It's quiet outside.

5th July 11:50am

Feeling a bit nervous about using my phone and wary of Kim plus I keep thinking that people are following me and that I am going to get jumped in the corridor and given a right kicking. So I walk fast and check over my shoulder if I think I hear someone. It's horrible.

3:45pm

Saw Den which was lovely but I had to send him away because after a while I was finding it REALLY hard to manage the noise in my head AND talk to him. I feel FUCKING TERRIBLE right now — on top of all the stuff about my phone, being scared of the staff and thinking I'm going to get jumped I'm also really WORRIED that I've done something AWFUL that I can't remember. Paranoia and self persecution SUCK. I think I am going to puke. I'm EXHAUSTED.

5:40pm

FINALLY fell off the paranoia boat and landed in the cool clear waters of rationality. My PRN works. That's all there is to it.

Physically I still feel quite crap — It's like I've been hit by a large truck: I ache all over, especially my neck and back.

I am NOT some PRN junkie and I will continue to bug staff for them BECAUSE THEY HELP. I know distraction techniques are important but hey, let's play "Spot the chemical imbalance!" When I don't have the right medication I'm like a diesel car trying hard to run on petrol. No amount of distraction techniques will make the horror show in my head go away — I NEED the medication.

6th July 9:30am

Last night? Hmmm. I DO know that I felt pretty damn great until around 9:00pm and it was like someone flipped a coin and everything went black inside my head in the space of a few minutes. I wanted to leave and hang myself. I think that's pretty much all there was to it. BUT it didn't reach the really bad stage when I get numb, focused and determined to do both of those things. Is it crazy that being detained is a scarier option for me than the prospect of killing myself? I guess that's just where I'm at right now.

I was KNACKERED last night and after all the bad thoughts I slept for 8 HOURS. 8HOURS!!! Bloody Hell!

12:20pm

Heard my name being clearly spoken again on my MP3 player. It freaked me out a bit to be honest. I don't like it and I'm not sure what to do, I mean, if my distraction techniques are starting to mess with my head how do I combat it?

I've been feeling as if there is a lead weight squashing my brain today. Nothing specific is happening and there's no pain just a VERY uneasy feeling that something is terribly wrong. I guess I'll wait and see...

7th July 5:50am

My brain is broken. Couldn't remember anything about last night after I got my pills, barring a few fleeting glimpses here and there. Maybe that's for the best. Maybe it's better I don't remember what I was thinking and feeling. Maybe I'm losing it. I just don't know.

I hate myself right now. No, I utterly DESPISE AND LOATHE myself right now. This is meant to be my best time of day and yet I feel cheated because I have this HUGE INVISIBLE SLEDGE HAMMER crashing repeatedly into my brain. Shit, I feel depressed. You'd have thought I'd have learnt how to deal with this stuff by now but, no, I'm thrashing around in quicksand and I can't seem to escape. And I'm scared 'cos suicidal thoughts are lurking. I've got to fight this because it's too fucking scary to let this win.

Feeling a bit better after a PRN.

11:58am
DIDN'T WANT TO GO.... but went anyway to Luss. Turned out to be a good idea and I felt a lot better as time went on. Got a bit stressed at the beginning (it's impossible to keep tabs on your surroundings when you're outside) but then Kathleen, the Occupational Therapist (O.T.) got talking about cats which relaxed and distracted me a bit.

Came back to the Ward and I went for an unsupervised 5 minute walk WITHOUT HEADPHONES and, y'know what? It was okay.

2:45pm
Doing good right now.

5:00pm
Grrr. Feeling shaky and I have this HORRIBLE feeling that something REALLY BAD is going to happen. Trying distraction techniques but I can't shake it and it's clinging to me like a very dark shadow.

7:21pm
Hugely suspicious of staff at the moment — any time they talk to me I'm sure it's some kind of test to do with a conspiracy

against me. YES, I have enough insight to realise I am being a tiny bit PARANOID but that doesn't make it go away. Took a PRN but it doesn't seem to be working. There's no one I feel safe talking to right now. WHAT DO I DO?

8:10pm

Feeling more relaxed because of 2 things: 1. The day staff have gone home. 2. Had a good chat with Katy and, okay, 3 things. 3. The PRN has kicked in a little later than normal.

...I'm Gloria Gaynor – "I WILL SURVIVE."

8th July 6:20am

After my paranoia-fest early yesterday evening things generally calmed down and I felt pretty damn good all night. I went to bed, for the first time in ages, with a clear head and NO paranoid/suicidal thoughts. Nervous about MDT with Dr Smith today though.

3:55pm

Feel like shit. Why does this keep happening?! Think I've got a grip on things at the moment but I don't want to write down what I'm thinking – it makes it all the more real and I don't want to deal with that right now.

5:30pm

Trying every distraction technique I know but the thoughts keep calling for my attention and tell me that a certain person on this Ward hates me. The suicidal thoughts peak and then SMASH ME IN THE FACE. And I can't find a way to get out of the way. I FUCKING **HATE** THIS.

10:29pm

Why didn't Dr Smith just say "No PRNs"? At least then I'd have known where I stood and maintained a semblance of dignity as opposed to my present situation where I have to constantly convince, justify and just plain BEG for one when I obviously (inside my head at least) NEED it? It's like saying to an epileptic "Sorry, that fit wasn't QUITE bad enough." And , yes, I'M PISSED OFF. Actually I'm ANGRY about quite a lot of things right now. Amongst them are the facts that when I am accompanied/unaccompanied the staff are spying on me and trying to figure out where my 'plan is located, my wedding has had to be postponed INDEFINITELY and that I can't leave the Ward at night without the threat of a Section hanging over me; apart from that and other things, life is fucking PEACHY. Oh yes.

What part of "Distraction techniques don't really work" is hard to understand? Okay, I concede they temporarily help when things are mild but they are as useful as a wet match when it REALLY kicks off. Right now I want to leave and that's my business. So leave it, please?

There is a place in my brain that is BURSTING with paranoia and if I casually stroll through, it sucks me in bewildered and confused. So obviously I try and stay away but the area surrounding it is sloping and slippy. I find myself unintentionally careering down into its terrifying depths and unable to shake off the persistent whispers and thoughts that lurk there. They coat my skin and eyes with a sinister film of suspicion and mistrust and leave me feeling persecuted and horrendously alienated from everyone.

Right now I feel as though I am being filmed and studied. THAT'S how I feel right now and I can handle it better by accepting it rather than constantly and exhaustingly challenging it. Is that so wrong? I have one life and I CAN'T afford to spend it fighting, FIGHTING, FIGHTING bad thoughts.

I just don't believe I have the resources.

I just don't believe in me.

9th July 9:36am

Have decided to ask for my PRN antipsychotic to be withdrawn. It's getting me down knowing that when I go and ask for one the chances are now that I won't be given one. So it's best to focus on other things and take the issue out of the equation.

10th July 6:40am

Tried going for a walk past my "Planned Place" in the evening but bottled it and came back early and a little shaken, but it was my first try so I'll cut myself some slack over that one. I figure that the percentage chance of me committing suicide has dropped from 97% to around 45% in the last few days. I STILL consider myself at risk so please can everyone, including myself, stay vigilant?

Got a bit paranoid about people walking behind me in the Ward, so PRN – less, I figured going to bed early was the best and ONLY way of getting away from it. Paranoia is NOT just in my head but covers my skin, eyes, nose, ears, mouth, EVERYTHING and it's fucking hard to rationalize it at the time and get away from.

Made a rough stab at playing Lydia my newest song, something I wouldn't have managed even a few weeks ago, so I really hope/think things are improving. Small steps though.

8:30am

Hmmm... just heard Katy say "Sorry Suzy!" very clearly when I was outside the smoke room... but I discovered she was round the other side in the clinic so I'm not feeling too happy.

2:50pm

Back from hairdresser — totally anxious and knackered though. Promised Ann something... shit why do I do this?!

4:45pm

Told Katy that Plan 2 was EXACTLY THE SAME as Plan 1. Anyway, she now knows the location and I have played all my cards. How do I feel? Pleased/pissed off/tense as Hell. I think I am improving (which is good) because apart from the voices and some paranoia at times today I've been pretty good. The weird (or maybe not) moment was that I REALLY had to fight off the tears when I was telling Katy about Plan 2 — that was TOUGH.

Katy and I are going to check out the site after dinner and although I realise this is an important step I DON'T WANT TO GO. Everything in me says "Stay the Hell away". I'm so dumb. How did I get myself into this situation?

...Ann!!!

11th July 9:10am

Do I look like a real person? Because I sure as Hell don't feel like one. Inside I died somewhere yesterday afternoon on my walk past "The Place" with Katy. Game over. My veneer of smiling jolly kept ticking along until about 10pm when it ran out of steam and mercifully gave up the ghost.

Yesterday afternoon and evening felt akin to a fine layer of shiny plastic floating on a pit of boiling, loathsome, GROTESQUE tar. The tar wins every time. There is no contest. Everything bad I know resides in that tar and it pours into my brain, my organs, blood vessels, bones, EVERYWHERE. How am I supposed to want to live when I feel like this. And why? FUCK THIS. Forget vocabulary, forget grammar and punctuation – what this comes down to is horrifically basic – I don't want to be here. But because I am a pathetic, winsome coward I will try to remember to keep breathing in and out and do my best to wait this fucker out and see if, when, somehow this gets any better. Just help me please.

I am throwing EVERYTHING I have at this.

11:40am

Suicidal impulses backing off a bit. Still feel horrible though. Why do I feel so disconnected and disorientated? I'm exhausted.

1:55pm

Feel sick from trying to sleep but not being able to. Still exhausted.

4:00pm

Trying to focus on new song and be POSITIVE with the lyrics – give myself a bit of a hammering on the chorus though. Still having bastard suicidal thoughts but they're not drawing my attention as much as before. Just focus on the damn song, Suzy.

7:35pm

I ache all over which is actually a welcome distraction from the thoughts so no painkillers right now.

Y'know what bugs me? How hard it is to have a space/a room/an area to yourself in here. People are around CONSTANTLY. Thank CHRIST for the loo and the shower which have locks. All right! Sanctuary!

Yes, I'm still making phone calls from the loo, thinking I'm going to be jumped in the corridor, thinking Kim has it in for me and destroying bits of paper because the info they contain will be used against me and... and... so on etc. But at least I recognise my paranoia – it's just that I can't STOP IT.

12th July 7:00am

Yesterday was all about existence. I felt that 'Suzy' had somehow disappeared and stopped being present and impacting. I didn't even feel as though I was in some 'tunnel' because I had no feeling of perspective or of being connected to anything. That included my family, friends, staff and fellow patients. I guess I spent up to 10pm pretty much wanting to end my existence on this planet. That's just how I felt. There was no great mystery or hidden depths to it – I just REALLY wanted to hang myself. But it had to be done in a certain place and in a certain way, both of which I had pre – empted myself by sabotaging. Killing myself on the Ward is not an option. There is WAY too much chance that I would be caught and be unable to complete the act. I'm not brave enough to be caught. I couldn't face everyone. So it's all or nothing for me and as such I'm VERY specific and controlling about how it's done.

However, my self preservation instinct and my friend, Ann are, as a combination pretty damn good at getting me to disclose resentful details of my 'Plan' ie the location and the means which PISSES me of greatly when I'm ill but relieves me when I'm feeling okay. I'm not playing games here it's just that I'm dealing with such contradicting thoughts and emotions (from day to day, hour to hour) that sometimes I'm not sure what I want or feel. Shit! And you wonder why I'm so exhausted and tense all the time???

Right now I feel okay – ish but the suicidal thoughts are ALWAYS there nagging and bickering in the background. When/how will this end? I honestly don't know yet.

3:51pm

Why is it that honesty and dangerous territory go hand in hand? FUCK. Okay, here I go, ah shit NO CONSTANTS PLEASE! Right at this moment I DON'T FEEL at risk but later/ sometime/whenever? I feel as though something in me has shifted and maybe not in a good way. Just now I feel I am staring down life's path to the horizon and looking tentatively at the view. I am standing perfectly still. But my logical brain worries for when the illogical brain takes over and I give myself the inertia and desire to leap over the edge. Realistically, things TEND to go pear shaped at night so as long as the door stays locked I should be okay. I REALLY don't want to get Sectioned either. You KNOW where the tree is and that it HAS to be outside. I'm doing EVERYTHING I can here to avoid all sorts of things, please recognise that.

7:35pm

Paranoid as fuck with the day staff after handing my diary into Katy – I have NO IDEA WHO HAS ACCESS TO IT! They all hate me and were looking at me weird. I felt very uneasy and threatened. Managed to get a grip by going for a walk with Katy and chatting generally with each member of staff. Bloody stressful though.

13th July Morning

I'm fucking STRUGGLING here. And it's getting HARDER.

ALL I can think about is KILLING MYSELF. Why? To shut up the dark whirlwind of confusion and despair spinning around my head at the moment. I DON'T NEED CONSTANTS but I DO NEED some helping hands to help me through this. This is TOUGH. That's all.

4:00pm

NOT feeling quite as desperate as I was this morning and it's now more 'phases' of black thoughts than a constant battering inside my brain. Someone turned the 'oven' down which is a relief. 70% convinced that the staff are plotting something against me which is stupid to write down here 'cos I'm giving this to Katy. At least they'll know I know. If that helps... kinda. I'm just niggled, not obsessed by it.

Haven't eaten today – too stressed – so having huge fucker of a curry tonight. Oh yes.

8:10pm

Just spoke to Lydia and felt absolutely okay. Cooooool. Suicidal thoughts are just quietly bickering away amongst themselves in the background so I feel pretty much fine. Long may it continue!

I'm not writing anymore today – I want to finish in a GOOD mood!

14th July 6:35am

Feeling okay this morning and quite pleased too because I slept soundly AND I slept soundly with EACH AND EVERY ONE OF MY SHOELACES, BELTS AND JEANS in the room! I was able to relax and NOT focus on them or have any suicidal thoughts kick off.

Unfortunately, got quite paranoid last night and was sure Lydia and Keith were bad mouthing me behind my back (plus I get pretty scared of Keith). The paranoia stayed at a low – ish level all evening but then REALLY SPARKED off after medication time and escalated. BUT. I was able to approach Lydia and question her about what I was thinking (didn't help though) and, although I had a bad dream, I slept well. So basically last night was, on balance, okay.

11:32am

Mood's dipped a bit and suicidal thoughts are starting to reassert themselves so I'm trying hard to block them. Heard my name said clearly 3 times in quick succession whilst I was listening to my MP3 player which was a bit disconcerting. There was no one around and I didn't recognise the voice. Strange, huh? It gives me the creeps.

Going out to lunch with Mum and Michel followed by a walk through Balloch Country Park with some staff and other patients so hopefully that will all be fine.

4:40pm

Just back from a LONG WALK!!! TOTALLY exhausted! Had a good chat with everyone but dark thoughts kept stalking me. I thought about running away... BUT I DIDN'T. So instead I focused really hard on making conversation and relaxing. Everything turned out fine so I think I did quite a good job — least ways I don't think anyone noticed.

We were all SO chilled at lunch and in really good moods — it was excellent. I saw a tourist wearing an "Alcatraz Psycho Ward" T-shirt and my suggestion of making a "I stayed at Christie Ward and all I got was this lousy T-shirt...and loads of medication" T-shirt to raise funds raised a few smiles! Progress indeed. I, as a consequence no doubt, stayed pretty relaxed and didn't need my PRN which I was VERY pleased about.

Felt paranoia creeping up on me when I went out for a 15 minute walk on my own — a bloke was walking behind me and I got scared and pretty certain he was going to jump me. So, what did I do? Panic? No. Instead I took Patrick's advice and stopped and pretended to tie my shoelace. The scary bloke walked past. I was okay. Cool.

15th July 6:07am

Felt in good spirits last night and aside from one shitty moment everything was cool. The "shitty moment" was a really strong impulse to hang myself when I went for a shower. The good news is that (obviously) I didn't and after a few seconds, successfully challenged it. Still, it pisses me off 'cos I don't understand how I can be eating toast and having a bit of banter with another patient one minute and feel like killing myself the next? I'm sorry to dwell on the negative but I feel this is important especially due to the unpredictability of it. Perhaps I should talk to Dr Fallowfield about it tomorrow?

MDT today and I'm really hoping for an increase in my 'freedom' to an hour's pass a day. I realise that things can get very dodgy very quickly for me but I've successfully dealt with everything so far and besides, I NEED TO MOVE FORWARD (small steps though) and tangibly prove to myself that I'm improving.

I'm NOT in Christie to drink tea and eat toast and socialize — I'm here to GET BETTER and if I don't try what's the point of my admission? The medication can only do so much. IF I get the hour's pass I intend to cover my back and plan and structure my time out as much as possible to minimize any vulnerability (unexpected thoughts etc). IF they happen I've got my phone and anyway I wouldn't be venturing too far.

PLEASE trust me.

1:00pm

Felt really nervous and emotional during today's MDT which was kinda weird. This 'getting better' stuff can certainly take it out of you! Anyway, the MDT, as far as I can recall went well: antidepressant up to 20mg, 1 hour time out and a free chicken korma (nope). So all is good. Gonna work on a relapse plan with Katy so I'm thinking about that.

Just returned from first hour time out armed with a chicken pasty and 12 cans of coke. Sorted. How did it go? Fine, mostly. Got a bit freaked a couple of times but I kind of expected that. My MP3 player was a BIG help as it cut out all the noise that goes on in town eg cars, people etc so felt less threatened and in danger.

Bumped into Katy who was holding a lasso and a stun gun (just kidding). Hmm...maybe I'm not paranoid and YOU REALLY ARE following me!

So all in all it went well — as well as I'd expected anyway, and as a consequence I'm feeling pretty chuffed with myself. As you can no doubt tell. The crappiest bit was that I've lost my ability to judge the speed of oncoming cars so after a close call I'll be crossing at the pedestrian crossings from now on. I do not intend to be hit by a car after all the shit I have been through. That would NOT be good.

4:14pm

Everything's FINE so why do I have a horrible feeling in my stomach that something BAD is about to happen. I feel sick and nervous but most of all I seem to have lost that feeling of SELF that I had back this morning for a while. The whole sense of who I am has been sifting through my fingers like dry sand for the last ½ hour and it's BOTHERING ME! WHY IS

THIS HAPPENING??? I feel totally disconnected and weird. My mood is okay, I'm a little edgy about a few things but most of all I'm just disappointed that I don't feel the same as I did this morning/early afternoon...and I am as impatient as a 6year old waiting for Xmas! I just want to feel like ME again.

I THINK the reason I feel a little bit strange is because for the last 7 MONTHS (since January) I have felt like UTTER SHITE, both mentally and physically, so I'm not USED to feeling good and it's taking me by surprise a bit! I'm so unused to it that I'm not sure how I'm even supposed to BE when I'm well so it's all a bit odd.

Does that make sense or is my brain totally GONE?

16th July 9:02am

Do birds EN JOY flying? Just wondering...

Feeling fine this morning. Went for a walk around 7:30am and got a bit spooked 'cos I was sure someone was following me for most of the way around the grounds. Turned out there wasn't.

Seeing Dr Fallowfield this afternoon and I have to confess I'm pretty nervous and NOT REALLY looking forward to it. I think memories of my previous experience (although not the same as it was with a psychologist) are haunting me and are doing their best to gain my attention. Oh shit (immaturity alert). Found out I have developed a pretty unhealthy fear of public transport but I'll sort that out much further down the line when I've been home for a while.

I guess I'm wanting to go home when I'm feeling okay and these spells are getting longer and longer. BUT, and it's an important "but", I can't afford to be discharged too soon. It would be CRAZY to blow it now and find myself at risk either of my symptoms returning or of suicide so I MUST be patient and give myself a bit of time and recovery or else the very real danger is that I'd end up back in here and, no offence to anybody, I REALLY don't want that!

8:11pm

Bearing in mind that I now REEK of garlic and korma sauce today has been a good day. The main event, next to Mitch visiting, was going to Riverview to meet with Dr Fallowfield. I THINK it went well... at least I got something out of it which I guess is the point. We talked fairly extensively about paranoia and the way it messes up your thought processes and my own particular thought processes gave an example of this when I became uncomfortably suspicious of a black glass box with a green flashing light on it that was attached to the ceiling. I was pretty damn sure I was being filmed. BUT the good part is that rather than letting the idea/thought build uncontrollably and basically do my nut in I voiced it (after a few minutes) and Dr Fallowfield very obligingly went off to get the janitor to tell him what it was. It turned out to be an alarm sensor. AND, because the paranoia hadn't had a chance to escalate and because I think Dr Fallowfield's a good guy and I trust him, I BELIEVED HIM! EXCELLENT! That more than anything else we talked about (although we talked about some important stuff) really cut into my brain and gave me some hope for the future.

VERY cool. Maybe I can beat this... if I address it early enough?

17th July 9:35am

Black is never so black as when it's sitting next to white. Do I feel depressed. I feel as though something has gutted me like a fish and all that's left is a dark, bleeding cavity where everything that is ME used to reside. YES, I feel depressed. I DO feel less paranoid than last night's "everyone is talking about me" fest and I'm NOT hearing voices anymore but, and honesty is beating me with a BIG STICK here, I am a bit preoccupied. Suicidal thoughts are ricocheting around my head like bullets bouncing off a steel door. I have them under control for the moment but their presence is a ghastly, grotesque, DANGEROUS reminder of how paper thin the balance between good and bad is for me right now. And that scares the shit out of me.

A trip home for the day (planned for tomorrow)? Probably a good idea but untested ground and so I can give no guarantees. Maybe I'll be okay. Maybe not. Maybe? I really haven't a clue and I'm too tired and brain dead to think about it. So I'll just float with the tide and wait and see what happens...

4:32pm

Tough day. Not paranoid (okay — a little) but suicidal thoughts and depression are caving in on me like a rock face loaded with dynamite. I fucking HATE this and I know I'm being totally unreasonable in wanting and hoping to BE BETTER AND STAY BETTER. Slipping backwards is as excruciating as rusty, polluted nail scraping down the inside of my skull leaving infected, seeping wounds in their wake. I don't feel suicidal right now but I have thought about it a LOT today and it's plaguing me. I'm so TIRED, both of this and because of it. Do I believe things will improve? There is no option — they have to or I'm not going to get out of this.

10:37pm

...and FINALLY some respite! Around 10:00pm sometime just after my shower the lead weight that had been taking great joy in crushing me to bits all day backed the fuck off and suddenly I could see, hear, smell, breathe, Hell EVERYTHING again! However, before I have an Enid Blyton moment let's get back to reality — the suicidal ideation still lurks mercilessly bastardizing my concepts of hope and a future for myself and Mitch.

I am constantly having to screen my thoughts to make sure that I don't start giving myself options...options that could lead me into desperately wanted/repulsed by and scared of situations that reek of self destruction and death.

I don't want to kill myself but this illness does. THIS HAS TO GET BETTER FAST.

I'm done in.

18th July 6:20am

Because I'm a bit better right now (who knows how LONG that will last?) my mind turns to other things such as "how long will I be here?" Days, weeks, months? I have NO idea. I DO know that I am TERRIFIED of being discharged when I am still vulnerable to HORRIFIC thoughts — both paranoia and suicidal compulsion. I know what would be likely to happen if they occurred (at this current level) and I doubt I would survive for long. It's

SO HARD when I can feel fine one minute and then awful the next! HOW DO I JUDGE WHEN I AM BETTER AND AT MINIMAL RISK TO MYSELF? It's a crap situation and I have NO IDEA how Dr Smith, the nursing staff and I myself should pace this. I just know that if risks have to be taken then contingencies have to be made and safety plans dictated otherwise I could end up in a whole HEAP of bother. Like I said yesterday – I don't want to kill myself but this illness does.

Obviously no on can guarantee my safety but when I DO go home it has to be with the BEST CHANCE possible.

Otherwise, what's the point?

7:09pm

So what did I achieve on my pass home? I made a cup of tea and went down town with Mitch and bought a pair of trainers. Then I slept. I was TOTALLY EXHAUSTED by the experience. This is all much harder than I expected. Forgot all about my PRN which would have helped with the 'noise' in my head which was present all day so that was REALLY SMART.

9:50pm

If intimacy is a delicate flower mine has withered and died in the suffocating blackness of depression and psychosis. I can kiss Mitch (briefly) on the lips and hug him but that's about ALL I can handle right now which is kind of ridiculous considering I am an-in-love-35-year-old and that Mitch is the man that I want to spend the rest of my life with. I love him, I trust him and I fancy him. None of those are an issue or in question. The problem is that I appear to be completely bereft of the ability to respond to him as I normally would. Which is crap for both of us. He understands, puts absolutely no pressure on me and, STAR that he is, stayed awake cuddling me all afternoon while I slept. But I am TERRIFIED that he will subconsciously think I am somehow rejecting him. I need to talk to him about this but first I need to sort out the reasons in my head why this is happening to me.

19th July 12:39pm

SO TIRED. Feel absolutely EXHAUSTED (moan!). Pretty sure this is a 'left over' from my pass yesterday. My brain is bugging me with paranoid thoughts all about the staff and I don't know what to do with myself as my distraction techniques aren't really working. How can 3 hours at home totally kill me? Got to stop now and rest a bit and maybe get a pizza ordered in this afternoon. Got to eat more...and lunch was CRAP.

20th July 5:50am

I had to fight REALLY HARD yesterday because the paranoia was taking a pretty full on hardcore grip. Everything peaked at around 6pm and I felt as though my head was going to BURST as it was SO FULL of negative, persecutory thoughts. Add panic to the mix and you might get a feel for how SHITE I felt. BUT... one PRN and an hour(ish) later and AMAZINGLY the thoughts gradually dissolved into the ether and FINALLY I could relax and breathe again. Does that mean that my paranoid thoughts are more physiological than psychological? I don't know. All I know are two things: 1. It worked WAY BETTER than my rather feeble (in comparison) distraction techniques 2. After about 3 hours I felt so relaxed and comfortable in my skin that, on request, I was able to play my new song in reception!

6:50am

Ah shit. The thought "...but it was a placebo." Is lazily rotating in my brain. I don't know when it started or where it came from but it's there and, believe me, it can FUCK RIGHT OFF. I'm too tired to cope with another day of paranoia so PLEASE BACK OFF.

9:50am

Feeling better. The paranoia is chilling out and enjoying the sunshine for the moment and mercifully leaving me well alone. However, the sound of the lunch trolley coming down the corridor is locked in my brain and set on constant repeat. It's not too bad though and better than bad thoughts any day.

2:40pm

Feeling pretty wiped out and vulnerable again. However, Mitch is due in an hour so that gives me something to focus on and look forward to.

21st July 6:05am

Felt UNBELIEVABLY tired last night and as a result 2 things happened: 1. I started hallucinating (visual) — insects as usual — around 9:45pm and felt as though the floor was moving. 2. I went to sleep around 10:15pm and pretty much slept until 5:45am. Still feeling a bit of confusion (for want of a better word) this morning and it's as though there is a lot of noise in my head. I have to put more effort into thinking clearly and making sense

of things which is a bit annoying (and tiring) but I can cope with
that and, again, hopefully this will fade.

6:40am

Just puked. Nice. I tend to be sick when I'm struggling physically
so it was kind of expected... (unless I can get pregnant from
holding Mitch's hand...).

8:32am

Uh... I have no memory of writing the 6:05am entry. Hmmm. At
least it makes sense to read and is not utter nonsense. Feeling
a little edgy but I'm doing okay and I find I can dampen down bad
and paranoid thoughts fairly easily.

5:25pm

Went for a walk with Pippa and came back knackered and
feeling as though I had been crammed into a washing machine
stuck on its spin cycle with only horrific thoughts as my companions.
The THOUGHTS NOT VOICES bombard me ceaselessly and
are impossible to manage in a head that feels pressured and
about to explode. I'm TIRED and trying to cope. Got my MP3
player back (it had been re-confiscated a few days ago) and
that has helped — the thoughts are still present and active but
packed a bit more into the recesses of my brain and not quite so
immediate and demanding — so I'm HOPING that tonight will be
okay. I'm trying to rest but that in itself leaves me vulnerable and
as I'm too tired to be active for long I am a touch worried about
how the evening will progress. I'll try and have a chat with Katy
about it and see what she thinks or suggests. I also worry about
falling asleep as that short period between being awake and asleep

is when the thoughts lose any inhibitions they might have had and attack and stab like NASTY VICIOUS THINGS. It's horrendous and I feel very scared and out of control. But I have to sleep so what can I do?

22nd July 6:45am

I feel quite depressed this morning which I'm not too surprised at given last night's events. I woke at some point between 12:30 and 3:30am and lay awake for a while certain that my bed had been relocated to reception and that 1. Katy and Miriam (one of my roommates) were talking about me just out of sight. 2. strangers kept walking past my bed and I only had my curtain to keep me safe. I couldn't read my watch properly and time kept jumping back and forth. All this time I felt sick and uneasy. I can't tell how long this went on for — it could have been 3 hours, it could have been 3 minutes — I just don't know and that bothers me.

I got up and spoke to Katy which helped re-orientate my head and fell asleep with a particularly special nightmare for company. (But at least I COULD SLEEP.) Woke at 6:30am and I'm knackered but more sleep is out of the question.

MDT today.

1:00pm

The MDT was disheartening. I think I was always going to be disappointed as anything other than "Take this pill and you will be fine ...NOW" would have fallen short of the mark. I AM SO FED UP AND DISCOURAGED right now. I HATE being who I am, thinking what I think and expressing things so poorly. If you could see through my skin (which I think you CAN at times) you would see that I am packed solid — in every crevice and inside every bone and blood vessel with filthy, contaminated, radioactive dirt. It walks with me, breathes with me and sleeps with me — there is no escape. Yes, I have times of relief but even then, when I am resting, the dirt rests too and recharges itself so that when it pours once again, choking my heart and clogging my brain, it is eager and ready to recommence its sick, fucked up assault on everything that makes me ME. I'm so TIRED of all of this and more than that there are times when I'm tired of fighting and want to, HAVE to, quit. I don't know what the consequences of giving in might be but to be honest I don't really care that much. I wish I could just be erased from this planet in a way that no one would remember me and no one would be upset. I could just STOP. That would be nice. I realise I am feeling extremely sorry for myself right now but I really don't like being in my skin at this moment.

7:31pm

Feeling a BIT better. Thank fuck for that. I'm now more angry and frustrated at how things are not progressing at the pace I would like than depressed and miserable. I just want everything to be NORMAL again. But they're not. Yet. It seems like "when" and "if" are the magic words at the moment. Bad news — thought a lot about suicide today, kind of alarmed myself actually. Good news — only very mild paranoia! Yeah! It was centred around Kim but after my 1:1 with her at 6:45pm it dissipated. She reminded me that when she's my nurse for the day and I want some time out off the Ward I HAVE to report directly to HER. How did that make me feel? Actually, watched over and secure which is good. Felt 2/10 earlier but up to 7/10 now. Cool, eh?

23rd July 7:03am

WAAAAAAAH!!! The fire alarm kicked off at 5:30am (at least I hope it did or else I had a pretty fucking impressive and sustained hallucination.) There is NEVER a good time for an alarm to go off but 5:30am is pretty special by all accounts and the bummer was that I was in the middle of a really good sleep. GRRR! And all because someone was having a barbecue downstairs...

Last night was MUCH better than the day had been although I was KNACKERED and had this horrible feeling of impending doom sitting on my shoulder taunting me. So what did I do? Take a PRN? No. Call Jimmy Saville to see if he could 'fix it' Nope. Panic?.... A little bit. But sensibly (I think) I weighed everything up and decided the best thing to do was to hit the hay and at 10:20pm I called it a day and went to bed. I slept really soundly and had no spooky hallucinations, at least until...

Feel okay this morning, a little paranoid, but okay. Hoping to go home tomorrow for a bit and I'm also seeing Dr Fallowfield today at 2:00pm.

11:56am

Paranoia still lurks and jabs but I'm handling it okay and am NOT in need of a PRN. Went out for an hour and aside from idly toying with the concept of hanging myself from a tree in Christie Park (didn't go in) it was fine and I felt quite pleased.

Suicidal thoughts DID bother me this morning but I'm not TOO bothered because 1. they were only THOUGHTS not solid plans with action and motivation behind them 2. I'm pretty used to them (which in its own way is a bit shit).

I think I'm realistic enough to appreciate that they're never going to go away completely. What I would like is for the intensity to decrease so that I can deal with them better and not be so scared of them. Plus, obviously, they impact on my mood, self confidence, self esteem etc at this level and I can do without that.

1:14pm

Have managed to talk to all of the nursing staff (except Caitlin and Simon) so I feel as though I am managing the paranoia reasonably well. It bugs the fuck out of me though. Anyway, waiting for Dr Fallowfield to arrive.

3:15pm

Hmmm. Dr Fallowfield gave me some food for thought. Basically my opinion that I am a totally shit person and the fact that my current situation is all my fault is equivalent to beating myself with a big stick and I'm giving myself an unnecessarily hard time of it. I just think if I was a better person I would be able to cope with everything and not have to end up in hospital and put my friends and family through all this crap. Also, if I was a better, stronger person I would be making a faster recovery instead of having pissy days like the ones I am experiencing. FUCK! I've never liked myself but even I realise that I'm throwing petrol on the fire and that my doubts and self hate are holding me back. The thing is that I don't know how to change. How do I change? Is it possible TO change? I've been like this for as long as I can remember. It's like this big anchor holding me back from 'what could be'. And what is that? Maybe it's 'happy' and 'better able to cope with my symptoms'?

THAT would be cool.

24th July 6:35am

It's amazing how well you can sleep in the absence of a fire alarm! Slept soundly from 12:30am – 6:00am and I'm feeling pretty okay thank you very much.

Actually I was feeling SO good this morning that when Katy and I had a chat in one of the doctor's offices and the phone on the desk began to ring I grabbed the receiver and barked "Yes? Dr Johnston?" down the line! I have NO IDEA what the person at the other end made of it all but I DO know that Katy nearly fell off her seat laughing and I had a tough job keeping a straight face.

I was really quite chuffed with the whole "Dr Johnston" thing as it was the first time in AGES that I have been spontaneous and stupid (in a positive and fun way) without worrying myself to DEATH about it afterwards. Progress, methinks.

10:25am

Paranoia is tapping me on my shoulder and casting a shadow over my sunny mood. Fuck. I keep pushing it away but it is like a poly bag half filled with water, unwieldy and difficult to manage. I have it fairly well controlled at the moment but distraction techniques are the order of the day and I must keep focused. Hoping to go home for a few hours this afternoon. I think it will be fine.

8:00pm

My afternoon pass went well and aside from a bit of nervousness walking along the busy front everything was good. Didn't feel confident enough to go for a walk on my own but at least I can visualize it happening at some point in the future.

25th July 6:10am

A big, articulated truck of suicidal and paranoia SLAMMED into my brain at around 9:40pm last night. It's so fucking unfair. I was washing my hands in the bathroom when the persistent, demanding and awful NOISY thoughts of death rang through my head. As slowly as I could manage I undid my watches in an attempt to block the urge to take off my belt. It sort of worked because even though I took my belt off next, the thoughts had backed off a bit, at least to the extent that I could handle them.

Paranoia is a horrendous thing. I was absolutely SURE that Lydia and Alice were talking about me last night and using a code made up of numbers and other people's names. I didn't feel safe and vulnerability and FEAR shrieked through my veins.

How on earth will I manage if this happens when I am living at home??? PRN? I was so preoccupied last night that the thought of taking a PRN never even OCCURRED to me. I was in trouble...but after talking to Alice (and having my belts, shoelaces etc removed) the symptoms backed off a bit. I just worry that I wont be able to talk to my family or friends about this stuff and I DON'T want to burden Mitch so WHAT DO I DO? **I HATE THIS.**

10:00am

I feel a bit better this morning but still a bit damaged and unsure about things so I have to protect myself and focus so that things don't get bad again. I'm going for a walk in Luss later so I will try and fill my head with thoughts of that. Right now? It feels like my head is broken.

10:30am

There is a big abscess inside my brain filled with bad thoughts. I've got it contained for the moment but it causes me worry.

2:05pm

Despair and depression choke me and fill my bones with apathy laden dirt. AAAAAARGH! God, I hate this! Have nearly been sick twice because of the revulsion I feel for myself. Too worn out and done in to feel paranoid or suicidal so that's not a problem right now. I feel isolated and alone inside my own cramped bell jar. Nothing feels real — people, objects, NOTHING.

4:30pm

I HAVE NO WORDS TO ADEQUATELY DESCRIBE HOW I FEEL.

5:35pm

I heard the dinner trolley rumbling its approach for about 20 minutes before it actually arrived. This has happened before and it's more disconcerting than alarming so it's no big deal. Got some fierce bad thoughts racing around my head but they're not "lodged" and dominating so I feel as though I can cope. Thankfully the depression has lifted a bit so I can breathe again and make some kind of contact with my surroundings. TRYING to stay focused.

28th July 7:50am

Doncha just LOVE fire alarms?!

Aside from that (and the strangely reassuring fact that doctors burn their dinners too — it's not just me) last night was okay. I even felt bold enough to play my guitar in reception again and another patient felt bold enough to have a shot too which was very cool.

After speaking to Alice I think I'm going to ask for a day pass for Wednesday and then an overnight for Fri/Sat just to get the lay of the land a bit better than just jumping into an overnight pass straight away. It's all up to Dr Smith, I guess.

Speaking of passes do you guys realise how fucking TERRIFIED I am of developing symptoms of the gravity of those that I have experienced whilst I'm here? I KNOW you're going to say "but you coped and got through them" but I really don't want to have it happen in front of Michel (or anyone else) and put them through what I go through. I'm worried that the safety factor will be diminished and that, if things are bad, the options are there for me to do something REALLY stupid. Of course, I KNOW it is up to me to handle things but I worry that I'm not a strong enough person to cope with this and that scares the pants off me.

Yes, I stayed out of hospital for 8 years prior to this but I still had to cope with shitty breakthrough symptoms. I guess what I'm worrying about is that what I've had to deal with in the past few months has been WAY worse and I'm just concerned about what could happen. I KNOW I have made it so far so I'm probably just panicking that there is a big abyss waiting for me. Realistically of course I'm going to have symptoms at home, I just have NO IDEA how severe they'll be. It's just something I have to deal with... SCARY though it is.

1:45pm
My hour's pass today was the best one so far — I felt relaxed and fairly comfortable in my surroundings. The best bit was buying a slush puppy (blue flavour — nice!) and NOT FEELING

PARANOID when standing in a monster queue of suspicious looking 'locals' (unfamiliar faces – kind of unnerving when you've been stuck inside with an assortment of around 40 people for a couple of months). So it went well and I'm quite chuffed. Oh yes.

4:00pm

I'm a bit/a lot worried about Mitch. He was giving a lecture at Cambridge Uni today (yes, he's WAAAAAAY smarter than me!). The lecture was scheduled to be 2 hours long and to top it all off he had a hellish journey down – stuck on an incredibly overcrowded train WITH NO AIR CONDITIONING for 9 HOURS. What a NIGHTMARE. Isn't it lucky that refreshments are SO CHEAP on trains??? Not. Anyway, HE HASN'T CALLED and his lecture slot was at 11:00am. I hope he is okay...

4:04pm

Obviously I have telepathic abilities that I was unaware of 'cos Mitch just rang and he's FINE. The lecture went well and he is... a living LEGEND – I'm so PROUD of him!!!

8:06pm

Why is it that I can be having a great day and then WHAM I have a visual hallucination of an enormous black beetle crawling across the face of the public phone. I HATE the unpredictability of all this. It's crap. Big time.

Clive has brought in his spare MP3 player for me to borrow until I replace mine. (I spilt orange juice on it... d'oh). Sometimes people rule. Nice one.

29th July 7:49am

I don't even know what to say this morning. I just know that I hate this illness. I HATE it so much that it burns my stomach lining and invades all of my senses. I don't want to live with this. I'm tired of struggling with it — it's wearing me down. Would YOU tolerate these symptoms — the symptoms that I am STILL getting even with medication? Maybe I'm not as big, bad and brave as I thought I was because this is really difficult and I fear for my future. I really do. I'm not being a drama queen I'm just frightened and worried that's all. And I think that's understandable.

In the MDT today I'm going to ask for a day pass and IF THAT GOES OKAY, an overnight (Fri/Sat) and stay at my parents'. I'm also going to ask for an increase in my antidepressant because I'm getting too many breakthrough symptoms which are of a severity that I don't think is acceptable. AT ALL.

5:25pm

Still feel a bit freaked out and vulnerable after speaking to Dr Fallowfield and I'm alarmed at how easily it happened. Hmmm. Thought I was tougher than that. Apparently not. Fortunately/ unfortunately I have a fairly good visual imagination and that can make visualisation tasks pretty fucking TERRIFYING. However, I understand where he is coming from it's just that every time I close my eyes or BLINK I see it again... and it's not pretty or big or clever. Actually I don't know why I'm joking 'cos I was scared. And I mean SCARED.

8:25pm

Just went for a walk and the weather is glorious – but kind of "could it BE any hotter?" in the Ward. Which sucks.

Feeling fine right now and hopeful of a good evening/night. There's even a new agency nurse on the Ward and I'm NOT freaking out! How cool is that?!

Avoided a horrendous paranoia inducing situation by CUTTING OFF a phone call to an electrical goods store that I had made to order my new MP3 player. I suddenly remembered how nuts I went last time – thinking all sorts of things – so I hung up rather than let fears such as "they're stealing my bank details" or "they're going to come and get me" take over in my brain. Wow, I think I'm FINALLY learning!

30th July 9:32am

Feeling A-OKAY this morning. If I'm being REALLY PERNICKITY there are some grumbling bad thoughts at the back of my head but, to be honest, they are always there so I guess this is what "normal" is like for me.

I'm looking forward to my day pass (and ordering my new cool MP3 player) and I have every confidence that it will go well. I'm also going to a martial arts class with Kathleen before I go home so that should be good.

6:34pm

Tai Chi (at least that's how I choose to spell it) was great and hopefully I'll go again next week. It was cool because it let me exercise without going all flat out/knackered like I do at the gym — being a competitive soul — and tempered my enthusiasm with controlled, deliberate movements. I lasted ½ hour which I was quite chuffed with as I didn't want to be tired for my pass — done THAT before.

My pass WENT WELL and although now I'm totally exhausted and a bit pukey all was good and I even organised Mitch into hiring a carpet shampooer for his house. I bet you're FASCINATED by that revelation. I even spent about 15 minutes alone in Mum and Dad's house and didn't think (okay, a LITTLE bit) about hanging. I came back to the Ward early 'cos I was tired and I didn't want to risk spoiling a good thing.

Oh yeah, NO PRN required! How cool is that?!

31st July 6:57am

Feeling fine although didn't sleep well — kept being disturbed (as opposed to FEELING disturbed — something I've done plenty of over the past few months). I'm idly wondering about my diary entries. My recollection of the past few months is a bit shady so I'm naturally curious. My only concern is that they could have a negative impact on me but maybe I am best to face and deal with that whilst I am in hospital? I dunno. It's not a big deal to anyone else but IT IS to me — I have to get my head around the "places" that I went/go to — horrendous though they are. Don't get me wrong, I DON'T want to dwell on them and get all morbid and miserable, I just want to exorcise these particular demons from my head and stop being so fucking scared of them.

It might even help my recovery? Maybe? Possibly? If I'm honest it's a bit of a gamble as I have no idea how I'll react...

11:44am

My 1 hour time out was not great because everytime I went into a shop I felt awful and sure that the shop staff were following me round the shop and talking about me to each other. I was okay on the street though, even when it was busy, but I nearly puked on the way back to the ward from all that tension and worry. Maybe events and behaviour on the Ward have made me more vulnerable today? I'm tired and there is a new patient in the Ward, Stella, who will not get out of my face and is a CONSTANT irritation. It doesn't take much to knock me off my stride right now so I must be selfish and think of ways to protect myself in order to keep the paranoia at bay.

4:35pm

At least the paranoia has dissipated but I still feel like shit. It's like someone's filled my head with 'white noise' and I'm finding it hard to think clearly. I heard another voice earlier, again saying "Suzy". It's not a big deal just a little disconcerting. I tried to sleep but just felt sick and it made what was going on in my head worse.

I think I've put my foot in it with Stella — she asked me if I thought she was fine and I replied, honestly, "No, I still think you're a bit unwell." Fuck. What can I say? She caught me by surprise and WAS NOT happy with my answer. Ah well.

8:32pm

Feeling MUCH better just a bit hot and I still have this white noise thing buzzing away which isn't a new phenomenon and causes me no harm — it's just distracting and tends to give me a headache. I think my physical problems were mainly due to being knackered from 1. My time out 2. being woken and kept awake by Miriam. From 4AM ONWARDS. Let's NOT have a repeat tonight, PLEASE!

August

1st August........

2nd August 6:50am

I know nothing. I thought that, by now, I'd be able to handle and control my thoughts but, once again, I feel like a boat adrift from its mooring. Yesterday SUCKED and, if I'm honest, I'm scared to bits about those kind of thoughts swamping me when I am at home. Mitch and my family are GREAT with handling my depressive symptoms but the psychosis seems to outfox us all. I know I have the relapse prevention plan but it has a BIG gap that I need to address — how to make my surroundings as safe as possible when I'm feeling like shit.

Last night was hard in that, later on, it felt as though my thoughts had totally JAMMED and I couldn't think or make even the most basic decisions about what I should be doing with myself — go to bed/ don't go to bed/hand in my belt/don't hand in my belt/hang myself/don't hang myself etc. It was complete inertia in my head and it felt horrible.

I'm still feeling a bit rough but I'm hoping for a day pass today. Mercifully, the unrestrained JOY of shampooing carpets has been put on hold so I just plan to chill out and maybe go for lunch with Mitch or something.

Anyway, I've had a good nights sleep so HOPEFULLY, once I wake up properly, I will find that I feel okay and that today will be better (I'm TRYING to be positive here!)

8:44am

Phew! I feel as though I have (mentally) FINALLY "exhaled" after holding my breath for fucking AGES. At last I feel as though I can relax and stop trying to catch and control my thoughts before they run away from me and mutate into something else, something AWFUL. Clive suggested that I phone the Ward from home during my pass today – just to touch base. I may, I may not – I'll see how things go.

8:10pm

My pass went well – slept and relaxed with Mitch for most of the day. The only thing that worried me was that I got increasingly ANXIOUS as the day progressed. About what I don't know but I'm guessing that after spending 4 months in hospital I'm bound to be a bit agoraphobic and anyway I think my social phobia was kicking off too. By the time I got back to the Ward I was shaking and ready to burst into tears but, somehow, I managed to keep it together. I asked for a PRN and since then I've just been trying to give myself some quiet time on my own to generally chill out a bit. It's hard though...

3rd August 10:56am

I felt SO anxious towards the end of my pass yesterday and that feeling spilled around my head kicking off the beginnings of psychosis. Even I could spot my early warning signs and, as I was beginning to feel pretty uncomfortable and horrible, I asked Gary if I could take my 10:00pm meds at 9:00pm instead of taking a PRN and then meds later. Fortunately he agreed and after about an hour I started to feel better and the bad thoughts backed off. I spent yesterday evening doing my best to chill out; listening to music and composing a new song – all very relaxing.

Today I feel knackered and worn out but otherwise okay so I'll just take it easy and hopefully avoid any problems.

I have this dilemma... is it better to approach staff and ask for a PRN to 'nip in the bud' any bad thoughts (right at the beginning) or do I have to wait until it is a tortuous, RAGING animal inside my head completely unresponsive to distraction techniques? I know which I would prefer I just DON'T know where that stands with the staff.

4:01pm

As I'm not going to take another day pass until after my MDT on Tues I decided to set myself a little task this afternoon – to go to the busiest place nearby and sit down and stay there for 20 minutes. So McDonalds on "Live at Loch Lomond" Sunday it was. I think I managed fairly well – I wasn't relaxed enough to read my book but as long as I could keep an eye on everyone it wasn't too bad. Obviously I had my MP3 player on which was a big help... and a cheeseburger and coke to distract me (naturally). Ironically, I think it would have been harder if there had been someone there I knew – conversation and all that – but luckily there wasn't. I guess meeting friends is the next step, outwith the safety of the Ward.

4th August 9:00am

I've got a dentist appointment at 10:30am today – feeling a bit nervous.

11:07am

All was fine and good at the dentist and my teeth are pretty much okay... so I guess it's time to crack open the chocolate and coca cola in the knowledge that my teeth aren't about to fall out or explode.

One of the weird things about feeling better is that my perception of the geography and interior of the Ward is TOTALLY different. A few weeks ago I would have SWORN BLIND that 1. My room was in a completely different place 2. The reception area was the size of a football field with tonnes of space behind the chairs and 3. There was a large foyer at the end of the clinic corridor. Strange, huh? I guess it was part of my psychosis.

11:45am

Feeling a little bit paranoid but nothing I can't handle – think I'm being talked about and the idea of a second set of notes has been floating around my head. Will play my guitar, listen to MP3 player and go for a walk with Kim as distractions.

12:00pm

Feel quite shitty and scared. Of what I'm not entirely sure. Very wary of staff.

12:30pm

Had a PRN. Went for a walk. Had a shower. Chatted to Ann. Feel like all of my hairs are standing on end.

1:56pm

Feel a bit more at ease and relaxed though still want to stay in my room and not approach or even SEE staff.

3:50pm

Still feeling nervous and concerned. This pisses me off royally because paranoia is SO debilitating and it just GETS IN THE WAY. Because of it, barring 2 walks, I haven't been out of my room today. I DON'T feel suicidal – just SCARED. I wish it would just SOD OFF and quit jumping on me when I least expect it. Kim just came into the room and a big bit of me was so sure that the staff have all been saying horrible things about me all day. So I know she's my nurse for the day and I should TALK about this but I'm STRESSED out and added to all my moans I have a killer headache. I HATE this and I wish it was night time so I could go to sleep.

8:56pm

Heard a voice whisper very clearly "Is Suzy there?" at around 7:30pm and I got that all too familiar sick and chill feeling. Hallucinations SUCK because they are SO unpredictable both in context and timing.

Plus they make me feel like crap.

5th August 6:25am

I think I want an overnight pass and although there is a whole bunch of crap grinding around in my head right now I'm still hopeful I will get one because, if I'm honest, I KNOW I'm going to get breakthrough symptoms WHEN I AM AT HOME and I have to find a way to cope with them.

How do I feel right now? Still depressed and kind of removed from everything and, yes, suicidal thoughts are lurking. I guess I'm still feeling a bit wary of staff which continues to irritate me. I'm trying to put these thoughts into a box and discard them but they are big and unwieldy and I'm finding it difficult to manage them. Hopefully, they will fuck off as the morning progresses. I'm SICK of this and when your brain is telling you to do one thing and, at the same time, suggesting the opposite, it is HUGELY tiring and confusing but I HAVE to learn to cope with this successfully if I'm going to make it at home.

7:34am

Feeling pretty isolated and alone right now.

12:20pm

Didn't get the overnight pass which I'm actually quite/very relieved about. The pressure's off and now I can relax a bit and concentrate on having a better week and successful day passes on Wed and Sat.

3:31pm

Quite anxious and a LITTLE bit paranoid after coming back from ASDA – mind you it was FUCKING busy, WAY too many people for my liking. Think I'll hang out in my room for a while and listen to some tunes. Feeling nervous of staff again, which sucks, but at least the 'disconnected' feeling has faded.

7:44pm

Just getting my head together after 3 hours of a foul psychotic episode. I felt as though my brain was a computer that had totally crashed. It was PAINFUL in the way that hearing a REALLY LOUD NOISE hurts – not physically but mentally. 2

things: 1. I felt all disconnected again – I recall holding Mitch's hand and not knowing whether I really was holding it 'cos I couldn't feel anything 2. I think this type of episode, whilst awful is an IMPROVEMENT in that it doesn't fully develop into paranoia or suicidal thoughts or any thing else for that matter. It just seems to JAM but fortunately it responds well to PRNs. I think a VERY quiet night is called for.

6th August 6:29am

Lydia sat and explained to me that a good way of reconnecting myself to reality is to focus on a really simple object eg an apple and hold it , smell it, tap it etc until my senses become a little bit more controlled. Sounds like a good plan to me.

I'm looking forward to my pass today; going to go to Tai Chi with Kathleen the OT, then go for lunch with Mitch and a couple of friends – so all should be good...although do you think it could RAIN any HARDER?!

5:41pm

I'm shattered and feeling pretty shaky. The first half of my pass was GREAT – went to Mum's, painted my nails, chilled with Mitch, went to the Deli with Pippa, Diane and Mitch but then when I got back to Mum's at around 2:30ish every sound became WAY TOO LOUD and Mitch brushing against me felt like BAD electric shocks plus someone had turned the volume up in my head and my thoughts were **SCREAMING** at me. Crap, really. So I took a PRN, waited for a while, heard a voice shouting "Suzy!" and thought "Fuck this" so I phoned Katy at the Ward and then came back over.

91

So my pass didn't go that well. Big deal. I still intend to go home again on Saturday and make it a success. That would be an even BIGGER deal.

7th August - The Sequel - 12:34pm

Lost my diary which, in a way, is a good thing "test – wise". What I mean is a month or so ago if I had lost my diary I would be going OFF MY HEAD with worry and paranoia – what if someone finds it and reads it?!! etc etc. But, let's face facts: it doesn't have my name on it, it's, quite frankly, NOT that interesting and EVERYONE knows Lydia IS the man from Del Monte (she said "yes" to me going for an extra long walk) anyway. So big deal.

The trip to and from Lomond Shores was fine and I even managed to walk past McDonalds without being sucked in the vortex and ordering McMy McUsual McMeal. So all was good and I felt quite chuffed with myself.

Note to self: try not to lose THIS diary. Fuckwit.

3:17pm

I've had a headache for a couple of hours now and that is the ONLY thing that is wrong with me so WHY THE FUCK DID I GET A REALLY STRONG IMPULSE when I went for my second walk of the day??? I put on my MP3 player, fought the urge to puke, placed one foot very deliberately in front of the other until I was back in the building and struggled with the compulsion to hang myself from a particular tree. Shit. I'm okay now – a little shaky but okay and I KNOW I should be focusing on the fact that I controlled it but it SCARES ME TO BITS.

How do I feel? Angry, angry that this happens. Angry and KNACKERED.

8:03pm

The compulsions I've just had to leave the Ward and hang myself were pretty strong (but not as strong as this afternoon). The trigger was glaringly obvious – the office was GLARINGLY empty and it would have been SO EASY... then May intervened and made the choice for me so guitar in the dining room it was. I'm sick, sick, SICK of this and added to the fact that its unpredictability worries me and scares the pants off me too. Plus I'm always shattered afterwards which isn't great either. Moan, moan, moan. Somehow I have to get my head together and start dealing with these suicidal thoughts more effectively so that they bother me less and cause me minimum damage and stress. Exactly how I go about doing that I am unsure. I really hate myself sometimes you know. I KNOW I control the thoughts I just DON'T WANT THEM IN MY HEAD, that's all. EVER!!!

8th August 6:40am

Felt fine yesterday evening – once the suicidal thoughts had pissed off – and slept well too. I'm going to take Lydia's advice and plan some basic tasks to help me reconnect should the depersonalisation thing happen again when I am on pass. Hopefully, now that I understand it better, I should be able to cope and, regardless of anything, I WILL HAVE A GOOD PASS (and a good visit to the hairdressers!)

7:26pm

My pass went WELL!!! Apart from some anxiety and bad thoughts (which I coped with) it really went well and I'm pretty chuffed about it. I went to the hairdressers ½ hour early so I could get used to my surroundings and chill out from the expected anxiety-fest that landed on my head. They made me a mug of tea and chatted to me, then I had my hair cut (jaggedly) with Mitch acting as my "holiday question bouncer" and I even coped with the "So what have you been up to recently?" questions by explaining that I had been occupied for the last four months by reading a REALLY, REALLY LONG book which had kept me indoors and out of sight (just kidding!) Seriously, I didn't want to mention the "Christie" word so like a big chicken I said nothing. And I got a wicked haircut.

8:46pm

I don't get it. I just DON'T GET IT. Am I missing something GLARINGLY obvious because I don't understand why, after a good day, I get the thought "You WILL kill yourself" belting around my brain like a game of Asteroids breaking up into more and more foul thought, idea, plans and fucking misery? It doesn't make sense — to ME at least. I HATE this SO MUCH. It's exhausting, crap, dangerous and I'm ANGRY WITH IT FOR ALL OF THOSE THINGS. I HATE THE WAY IT MAKES ME FEEL AND THINK. No one like being scared and threatened and this SUCKS.

What do I do when this happens? What I always do — PANIC and feel frightened and WEAK. No surprises there then. I'm TERRIFIED this is going to happen sometime, some day when I

WON'T be in a safe place with people around me. That scares the LIVING SHIT out of me. I HAVE to learn to cope with this BETTER.

Maybe this is how it is always going to be? What a fucking **HORRIBLE** thought.

10:07pm

I have this heart inside me that is made of lead and struggles to beat. Does time heal or does it just hide more unwelcome terrorists?

9th August 6:51am

I don't know where to begin. I have this TERRIBLE fear that my suicidal thoughts AREN'T GOING TO GO AWAY and sometime, somewhere — I don't know when — I AM going to kill myself. I KNOW I have been through some really horrible shit in this admission and, so far, made it through. I've had to be strong. I just don't know how I'm supposed to stay strong forever? I'm just not sure if I have the stamina. I realise that I will always have a choice it's just that sometimes, especially when I'm tired, I feel that I am on an escalator going DOWN and I can't seem to get off. I need help with this or this HUGE struggle that I have been through over the past 4 months will be all for nothing. Maybe I need to work a bit more on my relapse prevention plan? I want a future but this illness wants to put that future in a box and hide it under lock and key way out of my reach. I know I'm weak and feeling sorry for myself but I'm also ANGRY. These thoughts and voices scare me to bits. Fuck this.

8:01am

WHY do I feel like this??? At the moment I HATE myself and

I can't stand being in my skin. I could puke with self loathing. I can't put my finger on what's wrong — it's like a black shadow has crept across my brain and is blocking out the light. I don't want to dwell on this too much as it's doing my head in. Best to walk away.

11:30am

Welcome to my rollercoaster wilderness — could I have BEEN any more negative this morning?!! Thank God that gloom and misery has passed and I feel a whole lot BETTER. I think I used my distraction techniques pretty well — I wrote a POSITIVE new song all about Mitch, I made up some oh so life-affirming lists, read Glasgow Herald's letters page (Mum's got a letter in) and I read a chapter of my book. All of these efforts helped drag me back to a happier place of existence that I'm MORE THAN HAPPY to linger in. The thing I was chuffed with most though was that I did this MYSELF without any need of prompting. Fantastic. I'm giving myself licence to eat additive fuelled ' strawberry pencils' as a reward.

I may be sick later...

4:32pm

Back from my trip with Mum and Mitch to Clydebank — still feeling fine but a bit tired so I should be careful, rest and eat something 'proper'...hmmm...I feel a curry coming on — hurray for take aways!

Still worried about the thing in my first entry of today's diary — see I'm nervous of even mentioning it — but it feels a bit more distant and less immediate than it was earlier today. THANK GOD.

11th August 2:25pm

Maybe if I pretend I'm asleep and lie as still and as quiet as I can, the torment in my head will stop? I'm really struggling today and I can't seem to get a break from it. Even when I'm really asleep I'm troubled by foul, persecutory dreams of being eaten alive by rats and leeches and I wake up filled with fear and depression. Fear and depression and dread. That pretty much sums it up. Plus suicidal thoughts that I'm not even going to do anything about right now – I don't have the energy or focus. I can't be bothered. Kind of like how I can't be bothered to see Mitch or eat or be social or ANYTHING. Can someone PLEASE stop this SICK FUCK of a fairground ride so that I can get off? I'm so tired and I don't like myself much at the moment. I just want everything to run quietly to a peaceful halt. There is a horrendous GRINDING going on in my brain at the moment as though everything has jammed. It's a surprise to me that I can write as I am finding it pretty hard to talk right now. And the PRNs aren't helping much...

5:05pm

I feel horribly isolated and separate from everyone. It's like I'm continually shouting for help and no one can hear. I'm living in a vacuum. I wish I could just step away from myself and turn and walk away but I'm ALWAYS in my own company and I CAN'T STAND IT. Katy was sitting talking to me just now and I wanted to tell her how I hate myself, how I can't think clearly, how I wish I was dead, how I'm finding it hard to judge the passage of time, how I keep thinking I am someone else, HOW MUCH THIS HURTS and how my head is filled with poison. Instead I asked if we could go for a walk...

8:14pm

Getting more unsure of the staff as the evening progresses and I feel edgy and nervous around them all. I feel as though they are talking about me ALL THE TIME and it's doing my head in. Still horribly depressed. And I don't know what to do about it. I can't seem to speak at the moment so writing is my only outlet. I had blood taken today to check my Lithium level and liver function – I guess I worry a bit that Hep A is going to jump all over me again but it's not my main worry, no, my main worries are 1. How much I hate myself. 2. How I don't want a future 3. How I wish I was dead and that 4. The staff are plotting against me.

I'm so **TIRED** of all of this

10:00pm

Feeling better about the staff after chatting to them about random stuff. Absolutely knackered though.

12th August 8:16am

All I want is for this to STOP. I can't say much more. Maybe the pills will work – maybe they won't. Things look pretty bleak right now and I've had ENOUGH. No big deal really. No big deal.

2 things: 1. I can't be bothered with today's MDT. 2. I can't blame others for hating me. I hate me just now. Actually, It's not so much that I hate myself, it's more that I can't stand feeling like this and it just GOES ON AND ON AND ON.....I have NO IDEA when/if it will end. I feel so DISTANT from everyone and the suicidal thoughts just keep on getting **BIGGER**. I THINK I can

control them just now. Probably. My thoughts are confusing, dark and all over the place so it's hard to concentrate and speaking is a huge challenge which is why I'm writing this down.

11:31am

Can someone please tell me what the point is because I can't see one? The suicidal thoughts are pretty tough right now and I feel like I'm shutting down. Maybe that's a good thing because then the pain might stop. The staff and patients might think that I'm quiet today but in my head I'm SCREAMING as loud as I fucking can. AAAAAAARRRGGHH!!!!!!!!!

3:55pm

I feel completely alone. I am surrounded by people constantly and yet I feel as though there is thick Perspex surrounding me, cutting off contact with anyone else. This Perspex is shatterproof – at least, it's too strong for me – and not only does it shut everything out it keeps in my thoughts, causing them to rebound, ricochet and ridiculously magnify. Every time I lose focus I find myself visualizing TERRIBLE things over and over again. This is a terrible, tortuous place to be and I'm trying to find a way out but the Perspex and the thoughts are too strong and I'm not ME right now. I would really like to go for a walk with Katy but it's pissing down outside.

On a positive note the bad thoughts I was thinking about the staff have gone away, so at least I feel less stressed about approaching the office. Maybe this is a sign that... I dunno, I don't want to tempt fate.

7:51pm

Unbelievable. 2 hours ago I had all but decided to make a break for it out of the door, run away and hang myself with my studded leather belt BUT an hour after a good chat with Katy and a PRN I feel that my head is FINALLY clear and the glass walls have been removed. I can breathe again. And breathe in air that is clean and pure and not polluted and toxic as it felt earlier. Earlier EVERYTHING was wrong somehow and I was rapidly in decline and fast losing the battle with my thoughts. Nihilism padded noisily around my skull sending out echoes of death and NO FUTURE. But now my conversation with Katy and the PRN have been my David to the thoughts' Goliath and their death has paradoxically saved me from stepping a damn sight closer to mine.

13th August 6:52am

Still having crappy suicidal thoughts this morning even though I feel better mood-wise than yesterday. I feel as though life has nothing to offer me and that my future is just a badly fitting suit with psychosis and depression lurking in the pockets. I don't want my life to be like this — knowing that any minute, any SECOND I could find myself on the depths of a brain choking episode. I have no control over this and that alone, never mind the symptoms themselves, HORRIFIES me. I KNOW I have Michel and he's WONDERFUL but not even he can take away these terrors. I also know that the episodes AREN'T as bad as they were 14 weeks ago but I'm getting to the point where I'm not prepared to tolerate them regardless of how bad/less bad they are. I would rather not be present. You can walk away. I can't.

8:16am

I'm not even angry anymore, just tired and dispirited. I'm finding it really hard to talk to people again — especially staff. I REALLY want to dissolve and disappear 'cos I don't see any other way out of this. I realise that a lot of this is probably down to my period — things are always worse at that time — and this will only last a few days. But a "few days" feels pretty fucking ENDLESS right now. Kim's advised me to play my guitar and finish my new song as a distraction... and I can get my MP3 player back.

Ever been reading a book and jumped, accidentally, from the beginning of one sentence to the end of another and found that what you're reading makes no sense? That's what it's like in my head right now. I feel disconnected, hazy and depressed. It's crap.

9:28am

Just read my relapse prevention plan 'indicators' and they're spot on which I suppose is good in a bad sort of way.

1:02pm

Feeling marginally less depressed for patches, then rubbish again, then a bit better and so on. I'm so tired today. And moany (in case you hadn't noticed). Finished my new song, "The Hardest Thing", which is about doing what you can to survive the circumstances I've found myself in — even using negative emotions positively. I think my song writing is less 'grim' than it was which is, in itself, encouraging. (GOD, THIS DIARY'S BLOODY RIVETING!)

3:25pm

FINALLY feeling better. Knackered but I'd give myself a 6/10 which is not bad especially compared to this morning. Got a bit of a depersonalisation thing going on but I can handle that. Just feels weird though — I actually feel as though I am occupying someone else's body.

Will take Lydia's advice and focus on some basic tasks until, hopefully, it fades.

14th August 10:31am

Okay, let's cut the bullshit and get down to the nitty gritty — SHOULD I BUY A PAIR OF HAIR STRAIGHTENERS??? I LOVE it when I'm feeling well enough to let (let's face it) not exactly life threatening issues concern me! I feel as though someone/something has caused the vice that was squeezing the life out of me release and when I breathe now I can feel the oxygen permeate and cleanse my body ridding it of the filth and corrosion that was there before.

I dare to lose focus today because I can sense that the part of my brain that wields the terrible, AWFUL thoughts has been cordoned off and there are big, bad bouncers guarding it. But, like every horror flick I have seen, there is ALWAYS a crappy sequel so I guess right now my life is all about the present — this moment, NOW. I can't afford to be bitter about that or what is good right now could oh so easily melt and slip away. I'll deal with the future when/as it comes... I don't believe that this is pre-empting things in any way — I KNOW I will have horrible, HORRIBLE days, that's fact not imagination and I also, albeit rather morbidly, know that I am destined to commit suicide at some point. But, while that belief is still fixed, it no longer feels as immediate and compelling... at least not today... and I will live my life as best as I can, until it finishes – that's all any of us can do.

4:46pm

Just back from Jenners (and 100's of obnoxious children) and I'm pretty whacked. Feeling positive about tonight mood-wise and I'm hoping to go on a day pass tomorrow from 10:30 – 6:30pm and have a day chilling with Mitch.

8:25pm

The hospital kitchen forgot to put my dinner on the trolley. Bummer... I think that was most DEFINITELY God's way of telling me to order a take away. And I have since discovered the AMAZING recuperative powers of honey and garlic ribs. FANTASTIC. I'm also very pleased to report that Pam is back from her holiday which is very cool...

15th August 8:32am

I'm feeling a lot better but (there's always a but isn't there?) I'm hopefully not dumb enough to ignore the little whispers resonating in the dark, murky depths of my brain and be aware of them just enough so that I can recognise them but, at the same time, dampen them down and control them. I think, at the moment, I'm handling them well and they don't pose a threat to me. I'm pretty confident that today AND MY PASS will go well.

6:38pm

Today went absolutely FINE barring two small incidents which I dealt with. The day went something like a Robbie Williams song:

not much content and easy to fall asleep to and the glitches themselves were kind of weird – I went to the hairdressers and felt that for around 10 seconds the people sitting around me were speaking in some sort of alien language. I think it was that depersonalisation thing 'cos I felt a bit odd and really anxious (plus Mitch wasn't there). Glitch 2 was minor – just anxiety and agitation towards the end of the pass. But all in all I felt it went well AND NO PRN REQUIRED. So that's good. I guess the anxiety stemmed from the hairdressers and just got worse as time went on. But I MANAGED.

8:40pm

Damn. Speaking to Alicia about my pass on my return to the Ward was AWFUL. I wanted to die and for the clinic floor to open up and swallow me. I felt SO ANXIOUS AND MISERABLE and just generally SHIT. Christ, I even nearly started crying and I think she knew it. I was trying SO HARD to appear cool, calm and vaguely collected but I think she sussed and gave me a PRN. Why does this happen?

16th August 8:58am

Last night wasn't terrific, especially towards the end. I'm not that surprised though as I had been feeling mucho anxious all evening and there were BAD thoughts dive bombing my head and making a general nuisance of themselves. Pam sent me to bed, so I picked up my bloodied brain and occupied myself with distraction techniques – reading a bit of a book and listening to music – until I conked out. I slept from about 12:45am – 4:00am then 5:00am – 6:00am. I just feel so fucking ANXIOUS and I don't know what about*, plus I can sense a dark fog in the distance and I can't gauge whether it's moving towards or away from me. Hmmm. Better keep my guard up.

My intentions this weekend are to have a quiet chilled time on the Ward and get my head together a bit, ready for going out again on Monday. I just feel a bit all over the place at the moment and, joy of joys, my social phobia (fear of people) has come ROARING back into my life again. Terrific. How do I feel when it happens? Kind of like extreme anxiety and as though I am about to explode, implode and burst into tears all at the same time. I wish to God I didn't have it. (Moan a lot don't I?)

10:25am

*I've FINALLY figured it out. God, talk about not seeing the wood for the trees! The problem is EXACTLY what I've been whining on about for a while now — I don't SEE a future for myself. I just can't VISUALIZE one. I can't see, in my head at least and this sounds terribly melodramatic, or feel HOPE. Sure I can talk about it objectively and make all the right noises but, let's face it ladies and gentlemen, unless you FEEL it you don't have much going for you. Of course, I DO get fleeting moments where I feel okay and they're GREAT but my overriding belief as I have spoken about before, that I will kill myself at some point and I'm HUGELY CONCERNED that I will get discharged before these thoughts and beliefs have been properly addressed. I KNOW Katy helped me make up the mother-of-all-relapse-prevention-plans and that's a great start but, greedily, I just don't want to have these thoughts and overwhelming feeling of doom and stress AT ALL. Right now (10:35am) I have this

MASSIVE feeling that I often get that I have done something REALLY, REALLY BAD and I feel like SHIT. Suicidal thoughts are lurking just out of sight but I can sense them and they worry me.

6:25pm

I am still STRESSED OUT and anxious as FUCK despite a PRN and lots of guitar playing. I've STUPIDLY offered to play Lydia her song (She gave me three words: "Over The Sand" to write a song around) which is only adding to the anxiety(but I guess I'm a BIT proud of it) and whilst part of me wants her to hear it the other part of me is TERRIFIED. I feel so ill at ease, vulnerable, and nervous when I play my songs to people especially when I have to bloody SING: analogy – a half dead cat with a sore throat yodelling. Get the picture? At least that's what it feels like to me.

My social phobia is jumping all over me making it hard to have a conversation of any length with anyone (except Mitch) without feeling truly AWFUL. It's a real PAIN and I'm not sure how to address it. I have to confess that flooding techniques don't feel hugely appealing right now. So what do I do?

7:50pm

Suicidal thoughts bounce gleefully around my head leaving dread, worry and dull acceptance in their filthy, rotting wake. The greasy, choking liquid that IS my illness is seeping out of its container, oozing its way through the cracks and joins. It begins the very serious/sick business of coating my brain. I'm hoping to control it. I acknowledge its presence but it is NOT WELCOME HERE and I'm scared of its hypnotic and seducing powers. I realise that whilst I will probably win tonight there is a road in front of me and I can't discern its length because of the shadowy fog hanging over it. I am not very hopeful of my future. And I think that is a real concern and neither obsession nor nihilism.

17th August 7:47am

I can't even think properly this morning. All I know is that 1. I am sick, sick, SICK of feeling like this and 2. I want it to stop. For good.

I was planning dangerous things this morning but Katy said "No" to my feeble attempt to go for a walk so I guess I'll need to bide my time. It feels as though bad things are swarming around me like nasty infected horse flies, full of the worst intentions and poisonous to the core. It takes energy to fight them off and I'm TIRED. I'm lost in all this and all I want is a way out and some quiet in my head. I think I need it. Katy had a chat with me and then decided I needed a PRN so I'll need to wait and see if that helps... it's such a small looking pill though and it feels like it needs to be BIGGER. I suppose I'd better go and get my breakfast and my other meds. Maybe I'll get out for a walk later?

10:25am

Feeling a whole lot better, thankfully, and the "rope around my neck" sensation that had been stalking me since I woke up has mercifully gone away. Well, I guess the PRN worked. Nice one. Now I feel I can start my day properly without all that crap swimming around in my brain. When I'm feeling like that decisions are SO HARD to make so when someone asks me a question like "Do you FEEL UP FOR A WALK?" I find it impossible to answer and so I'm left standing there in silence like an idiot. The reason? I just have NO IDEA what to say and I can't seem to get any words out. Everything jams. EVERYTHING.

3:26pm

Guess what? Coke Zero tastes better out of a can? Asda sells sparkly earrings for £2? I'm feeling pretty damn fine thank you very much? Actually, all three are absolutely correct and, as sparkly earrings are a PRN in themselves it's not to be wondered at that I'm doing okay.

Mitch, however, is a bit subdued and I'm worried about him — he's lost quite a bit of weight since I've been in hospital and, whilst he's still healthy, I think I need to keep an eye on him. He's having a tough time with his Mum who is 86 and in failing health.

I spoke to Katy about how I'm doing with regard to the possibility of an overnight pass — which is a scary prospect but not necessarily an insurmountable one. Unless I am once again a shambling mute like last week, I will talk to Dr Smith about how I'm doing generally, my expectations for the future and the situation regarding passes. Things have GOT to be done slowly, NOT because I am dragging but because if I take too many big risks the chances are more likely that I will fuck up and that could have major impacts. Rushing things is NOT ACCEPTABLE. I NEED to have a secure and confident structure and bank of experience in place for me to stand any sort of chance of making it at home. Really. Because anything else scares the pants off me. Big time.

7:30pm

Two things 1. Got very paranoid at dinner tonight. Katy was on duty in the room and came after me in about... oooh... A SECOND when I had legged it out of there. We talked about it for a while until I had calmed down and then I told her the other thing – 2. There's an agency nurse who freaks me out and I would REALLY appreciate it if she was NEVER assigned to work with me. She's just in my face too much and CONSTANTLY tries to engage me in conversation which pisses me off. Harrumph. Ah well.

18th August 8:43am

Feeling pretty great this morning and looking forward to my pass. What am I hoping for? Straightforward with no unexpectedness would suit me just fine. Anyway, hopefully all will be good and I will return all smiles and ready to ask Dr Smith for an overnight pass later in the week.

9:07pm

RUBBISH DAY. I've had this strange noise battering around my head all afternoon and evening and it's still there despite a PRN. I'm SO WORRIED about Mitch at the moment – his Mum's ill health is really affecting him. I would probably have come back earlier from my pass (around 4:00pm) but I wanted to be with him 'cos he needs me right now. This is a NIGHTMARE for him. And me? I keep thinking about a particular tree and try as I might the thought won't shift. I've tried eating assorted crap, playing my guitar, having a shower, listening to music but I find myself focusing more and more on BAD things and this fucking noise won't leave me alone.

19th August 6:37am

It's too much. It feels like there are boulders raining down and Mitch and I are tied to a stake and we can't get out of the way. I still have this NOISE rattling about in my head and what with that and everything else I feel pretty ragged. Would I try and kill myself? Right now that question is the most straightforward thing in my brain at the moment. I'm SO TIRED of things being crap. I just want everything to stop. Please. PLEASE. I'm finding it REALLY hard to keep things together and Mitch is struggling too. I know I should be strong but maybe I just CAN'T right now. I feel as though I am careering down the side of a rocky mountain bruising and cutting myself on the way. And the thing that lurks at the bottom is dark and knows EXACTLY how to play me. I don't stand a chance.

7:41am

My walk this morning was CRAP and I ended up coming back after 5 minutes because it was like someone had drawn a highlighter pen over all the mess in my head and it was pretty overwhelming. I considered "The Tree", rejected that, then seriously thought about hopping on the bus to Glasgow just to give me some space to think about everything. Even I realised that was probably not such a hot idea. I'm trying to run away from myself but I keep catching up. Fuck.

1:15pm

The thoughts and the noise in my head backed off after lunch so I went for a wander around the Outlets and had a chat with my Mum (on the phone) about Mitch's Mum. She realises how much pressure this whole situation is for both Mitch and me. I have to confess it was good to hear someone else suggest that respite care was now required. I have to be able to bolster Mitch and I can't do that when I'm ill and if I became ill on an overnight pass — which is fairly likely at the moment — it would impact negatively on both of us which is the LAST THING we need. So, the decision to stick to day passes was a good one and I intend to go out on Thurs and Mon. I'll just need to help deal with Mitch's Mum and hope that, with Mitch's help, I can cope.

3:05pm

Feeling okay. A bit paranoid though that the staff are saying awful things about me and as a consequence I'm feeling kinda scared of them.

The session with Dr Fallowfield was good although I was a little suspicious of him which I think he picked up on because he volunteered to read out what he had written in my notes which had been quietly freaking me out!

I'm going for a walk now to clear my head.

20th August 11:26am

I'm okay today. Not spectacularly 100% but 'okay' and that's good enough for me especially as The Health Secretary is coming to the Ward today. Note to self: try and appear sane — no dribbling or twitching if possible. Seriously, it's GREAT that she's coming and hopefully we can all focus her mind on the job of saving Christie.

I went for a walk into the Vale and, as always, passing the treetastic Christie Park summons bad feelings and dark thoughts of hanging but I felt I dealt with it pretty well and was able to get past it to do some shopping.

I have NO IDEA how I'll be this afternoon, I just hope everything will be cool...we'll see...

5:16pm

Spoke... well actually stammered and shook a lot to The Health Secretary this afternoon in Patrick's office. I tried and hopefully succeeded in putting across how HUGELY important the Ward and its staff are with regards to its patients' recovery. This particular patient is WELL AWARE of how compassionately she has been handled over the past months and although meeting The Health Secretary was as nerve wracking as Hell, I felt I owed the staff one and MAYBE I helped a little today. I hope so anyway.

Feel absolutely KNACKERED now and have that white noise hissing round my head which is quite irritating and distracting (but probably not to be surprised at when you realise how STRESSED I was earlier).

Why are important things always so HARD to do?

8:32pm

Feel rubbish. The white noise continues despite the best efforts of my MP3 player and now I'm hugely worried that the staff all hate me because I spoke with The Health Secretary. I'm NOT paranoid. Una especially is throwing me bad vibes and I'm scared of her. I KNOW I should approach them and find out what the problem is and how best to sort it out but I'm DONE IN and feeling CRAP. Today took a lot out of me and I can feel bad things building in the back of my head and my defences are weak.

This is not good.
At all.

21st August 9:28am

Feeling kinda shattered both physically and mentally today – I think directly as a result of yesterday's STRESS. Still got that noise in my head but thankfully to a lesser extent which is a relief (but still irritating). I've decided not to go on pass today and hopefully go tomorrow and have a nice, chilled day with Mitch.

Last night SUCKED. In retrospect I realise that I was WELL paranoid and freaked out but I think the decision to get my meds early and go to bed at 9:30pm was a good one. Frankly, my mental state was just going to get worse and worse so taking a PRN as well as my regular meds was the best move and sleep saved me from a whole lot of grief. Hopefully today will be fine but I HAVE TO BE CAREFUL.

10:05am

Worried that everyone, especially staff, are saying horrible things about me... OR thinking them and not saying anything to my face. FUCK. I HATE this. It's doing my head in. I'm trying to relax but the fear KEEPS GROWING. I don't know why I put myself through things like yesterday. Am I some kind of idiot? Situations like that always mess with my head afterwards but I guess it was important and down to me to speak. No pressure then.

3:02pm

Shit. Felt a LOT BETTER after PRNs and a sleep but now? Now my brain is like a tiny piece of old, fragile china with cracks fast appearing in it. Paranoia is a tiny hammer tap-tap-tapping away causing the cracks to multiply and spread. I feel scared and suspicious of everyone. They're plotting against me. They're not. They are...they ARE. Confusion and doubt reign. A woman threw me a dirty look on my walk. Maybe she's having a crap day. Or maybe she's heard bad things about me and thinks I'm scum. Shit. I'm TIRED of this and need some help but I'm NERVOUS of approaching the office. I'm tying myself in knots here and they keep pulling tighter and tighter around me.

5:30pm

It's safest if I stay in my room. That way I can keep an eye on the door and see who's coming in. It's just safest that way.

8:33pm

Aaaaah... it's AMAZING how much a PRN can take away the confusion, fear, worry and distress of paranoia – along with a portion of honey and garlic ribs (natch!). Anyway, I'm feeling A LOT BETTER and as I've managed to talk with and feel comfortable around all of the night staff I'm pretty confident of a good evening/night. Oh yeah, and I am now, as dictated by Gary apparently, in charge of watering the Ward's plants. Marvellous.

22nd August...

23rd August 7:10am

I'm okay this morning — a little fragile and tired but okay. I moaned my HEAD OFF to Pam last night but in a way I'm glad I did because I managed to voice a whole load of worries that have been circumnavigating my skull for a while now eg. Why have I seemed to have reached a plateau in my recovery? Why am I still getting so many terrible symptoms? I'm worried because living from hour to hour not knowing how I'm going to be is NOT GOOD and I'm finding it impossible to envisage a future. That sounds terribly melodramatic I KNOW but I can't help that right now.

And then there's the worry of Michel's Mum...

8:01am

Going for a walk in the morning is usually a good idea but today it became a BAD ONE. Half way round I started to become consumed by BAD THINGS and... y'know what? I'll talk about this later 'cos I'm feeling a bit crap right now.

10:10am

I CAN'T SEE A GOOD WAY OUT OF THIS. The PRN Caitlin gave me has helped a bit but it feels like a very thin veneer holding back an ocean of negativity. I don't know how to win this. And I don't know what to do. I guess I have to put my faith in that veneer and hope that it holds. If it doesn't...if I write down what could happen it makes it more real so I won't.

I spoke to Mitch and said I'd decide about seeing him today later on. Which is a shitty way to treat someone. I KNOW that I'm tempted to push him away when I feel like this but I feel as though I'm in a monster battle with myself at the moment. Maybe I'll call him later. Maybe.

I want to go to the canteen for some cereal but I can see monsters the second that door opens and I don't feel as though I can trust myself right now — which is crap really, isn't it?

1:54pm

I'm less stressed but DEPRESSED and HATING it. Hating me. Hating my existence. Feeling sorry for myself aren't I? YUP. I'm desperate for these thoughts and feelings to GO AWAY but they are insidious and sneaky and keep grabbing my attention when I lose focus. I feel as though I am made of clunking, rusty metal and there is a big black, sinister magnet steadily pulling me towards it. I don't know how to stop this 'cos I'm just not that strong or brave. At all. And everything seems awfully DARK and SCARY. I'm pathetic and ridiculous and I SHOULD BE ABLE TO HANDLE THIS BETTER.

7:14pm

Sometimes it is better to keep things to yourself for fear of "consequences" ie constants. Please, and I'm begging you here, DON'T PUT ME ON CONSTANTS OR GET A DOC DOWN TO SECTION ME! I would LOVE to be able to give guarantees that I will not try anything untoward. I can promise you this though — I will not try anything on the Ward. All of my plans are based outside so if the door remains locked I am safe.

It's SO HARD because part of me is DESPERATE to leave and get it over with whilst the other part is TERRIFIED of that happening. I'm tired, confused and generally messed up and 'punishing' me for these thoughts would do more harm than good... THAT I can guarantee you.

Caitlin gave me some of her crackers and cheese for dinner because I had forgotten all about eating today — it just didn't seem that important. Phoned Mitch (briefly) just to say that I'm not in a bad mood with him or anything. I wish this was over. Depression turns my blood to poison.

MP3 is out of charge. Fantastic.

24th August 7:41am

Not sure how I feel this morning as I'm kind of numb. At least that's better than last night which was AWFUL — paranoia, depression and suicidal impulses. I felt as though EVERYONE had it in for me and I couldn't trust ANYBODY. It was a pretty horrible place to be. I was scared of the rest of the patients and SURE that the staff were thinking/saying terrible things about me AND secretly plotting to put me on constants (which DIDN'T happen).

Slept well though — not surprised because I was KNACKERED. How many times do I have to scream I HATE THIS?!! I couldn't even go for a pee or brush my teeth because I was scared of the suicidal thoughts that might be lurking in the bathroom. I don't want to kill myself but, damn, those thoughts DO.

I think I need to sleep and rest today if I am to stand a chance of making it out on pass tomorrow. Still don't want to see or speak to friends, family or Mitch which isn't great I know. It's still early though so I have some breathing space.

9:15am

It's amazing how matter of fact you can become about suicide. I'm trying to be open here so PLEASE DON'T PUNISH me for it. I feel safe indoors but outdoors is a whole other kettle of fish. I guess in my darkest moments the question that I'm faced with is: if someone has always sought oblivion how much of a TRAGEDY is it when they ACHIEVE that goal? I'm NOT saying I am going to kill myself right at this instant – I feel more depressed than suicidal at the moment – but I have to live with a time bomb in my head right now and I don't know how long is left on the clock.

I LOVE Mitch, my family and my friends but those emotions wither and fade in the presence of the thoughts that I experience. I can't help that.

I'm full to bursting with contradictions at the moment – call Mitch/don't call, speak to Caitlin/don't speak to her, go for a walk/not safe to, lose/win, breathe/don't breathe etc.

Maybe I should ask Caitlin if she'll go for a walk with me – which makes me feel like a five year old but if I'm honest I don't feel safe on my own so it's my only option.

10:55am

I've got something to say but I'll be damned if I can get the words together. Why can't I articulate how I feel VERBALLY? I feel SO inept and it's frustrating as Hell. Yes, I WRITE things down but I feel so crap at times that I honestly think I'm going to vomit with the strength of all the muted emotion inside of me. That goes for crying too. Must. Not. Cry.

Sometimes it's like the spoken word is a foreign language that I haven't learned yet. Sure, I can SPEAK but it's finding the words to express myself with that I'm having trouble with. This leads to a lot of awkward silences and I want to curl up and die. It's a real fucker and I feel like a stammering IDIOT.

3:46pm

If I can't stop myself maybe YOU can. That, ultimately, is the reason I told Caitlin 2 methods for hanging yourself in the bathrooms. Neither is rocket science but both are options I have considered in the past. All my options are now outdoor based so IF I stay indoors or am only allowed time outs when I'm in a good frame of mind (my responsibility as much as anyone elses) I should be okay (although not exactly what you would call either happy or comfortable).

Tomorrow's pass has been withdrawn which relieves me of a weight I didn't know I was carrying and I feel a little more relaxed. Can I save myself from myself? Right now I'm honestly not sure but hopefully by being open and honest you will all at least know I'm trying.

8:05pm

Caitlin spoke to Mitch and Mum which takes the pressure off me. Am I emotionally distancing myself from them? Probably, but I can't help that right now. Everything in me is telling me to sever contact with EVERYONE so I can be alone until I make up my mind as to what the HELL I'm going to do. I need time and space and NO distractions. But I can't THINK properly and it's doing my nut in!

I'm finding mealtimes really hard — too many people all around with knives and forks in a small room with only one exit. And you wonder why I get paranoid! So I didn't eat today but had a cheeseburger around 7:00pm when the room was empty and with the lights off (so no one could see in). Not sure how to beat this one. I'll figure something out.

Maybe.
Or I'm going to starve.

25th August 8:15am

I just wish I could step away from myself for a while and have a break. I wish I had courage. And motivation. This isn't ME —just a shell filled with crap and shadows of what used to be. And you know what? I HATE it. I need to fix this but I don't know how to. Please don't give up on me 'cos I'm REALLY TRYING not to give up on myself. I feel like I am a truly TERRIBLE person but I have NO IDEA what I've done...I don't even see the point of handing in this diary at the moment — what good could it possibly do? Maybe I don't want to let anyone in today...or tomorrow...or...

10:39am

The suicidal thoughts come in waves — pretty big, bloody monster waves at that — but for the moment they've backed off and, although depression still lurks, I can handle things—my posture is better, I don't shuffle or mumble and I can look people, if not in the eye, at least in the face (Kim told me about all this). I don't feel as though I have to control every thought and movement in order to prevent myself from running off the Ward and hanging myself. I don't know what I am doing but so far it has worked and I'm still here. How long this respite will last I have NO IDEA — seconds, minutes, hours? All I know is that I have to live like this for just now like a punch drunk boxer who doesn't know where the next punch is coming from. The thing is that my bruises don't show and I figure there's STILL a Hell of a fight in front of me.

12:15pm

It's frustrating how I'm unable to articulate how I'm feeling. The best I can come up with is that it feels as though all of my thoughts and emotions are one MASSIVE UCI cinema screen with surround sound and all of my senses have been superglued to it with volume, brightness and contrast all set on MAX. I can't get away from it and it's all TOO BIG for me to manage or make sense of. I'm overwhelmed. If I could just find a way to back off then MAYBE I could contextualize and cope a bit better. Today's "show" is abstract, bleak, noisy and seems to make NO SENSE. I'm TOO CLOSE and whilst TO YOU my problems might seem straightforward and easy to manage (do they?) TO ME they are baffling and impossible. The good news is the PRN seems to have muted things a little.

1:35pm

Just phoned Mitch, Mum and Dad to apologize for being a prize shitbag. Not ready to see them yet so stalled on that one. I

THINK I'm feeling a bit better although I'm still wandering aimlessly around in my "tunnel" with ABSOLUTELY no idea as to where the light is.

Sometimes I want to kill myself so much I can taste, smell and touch it BUT there are times of respite now peeking in through the cracks and though they are temporary at least it's something. I HAVE to cling onto that because its those moments I am dragging myself to like a shipwreck victim desperate for an island regardless of contents. ANYTHING is better than the dangerous waters I find myself thrashing about in at times. Anything.

7:30pm

Feeling numb and disconnected. Depression steals the life out from underneath you and leaves you with a gaping, hungry chasm that used to be where YOU used to reside. There's nothing to be done right now, at least. Must eat some food — just had a yoghurt today. I'm exhausted.

26th August 7:18am

Got my MDT today so I'd better get it together enough to actually speak to Dr Smith. Speaking is difficult because it involves interaction with another person and I'm finding that hard just now. I feel really depressed this morning and it HURTS. I'm such a fucking moany coward it's ridiculous. Everything feels like it's MY FAULT. I'm not even feeling suicidal right now — I simply can't be bothered and I'm too numb to go there. I just want to sleep and not be present. Got to get through this. Got to. Apathy is a tightrope keeping me safe at the moment, I can't afford to fall off 'cos I'm not sure if there's a safety net. Monsters lurk in the shadows and LAUGH at me.

10:40am

Took a PRN about a couple of hours ago which helped and the MDT went well. I hope the medication increase helps because things, on the whole, are quite shit at the moment. I'm NOT going to get all melodramatic about how I feel suffice to say I'm struggling quite a lot just now and it SUCKS. HOWEVER, for the moment I'll give myself a "chunky" 6/10 which is pretty good considering how the last few days have been.

Mum, and Mitch are picking me up at 2:00pm to take me to see Dr Fallowfield in my home town's Infirmary so I shall see how that goes...

1:11pm

Buses are from HELL. They are. They rush up behind you all noisy and blustering, interrupting the breeze and smelling of dirt and almost certain death. I fear buses. No, I FEAR the impulses that sweep across my brain telling me, TELLING ME to step off the safety of the pavement and meet the insistent vehicle just like it wants me to in a no ticket required head on mess of me and steel. I WON'T DO IT. I couldn't do that to the driver or the passengers never mind Mitch or my family. But WHY do I have to put up with these thoughts and visualisations? I REALLY DON'T WANT to jump in front of a bus (or a car for that matter) but how do I stop the thoughts??? Maybe I'll talk to Dr Fallowfield about this... maybe.

5:06pm

I should wear a big sign brandishing the words "Not Brave Enough Today" because I chickened out of telling Dr Fallowfield about the bus thing. Ah well. Maybe tomorrow will be easier than its yesterday? Who knows? Certainly not ME as I don't have the first CLUE as to how I'll be then. Unpredictability SUCKS.

What Dr Fallowfield and I DID talk about were my, and I use the word loosely, "heroic" drives to do what I perceive as the greater good (hello Plato) with little regard for my own health and safety. I guess when you've had around 15 concussions this starts to make some sense.

But what he was driving at more were the consequences I had to endure when doing things like speaking to The Health Secretary which might have helped things for the Ward but REALLY SCARED ME TO PIECES. I KNEW I would pay a price for it but, even in my book Sat — Mon were hellishly BAD. So. He's going to help me learn the "N" word (NO) and try and start to get me to weigh up what's realistically within my capabilities and what I should say "No" to. For example, if I had still been in Ward 6 suffering from acute Hep A and barely able to walk, would it be acceptable to be told that if I went and ran 2 miles it would MAYBE help save the hospital? Hmmm. Honestly? I would probably have put my trainers on...

But that's just me. Maybe ME needs to change. Maybe the "greater good" is called that for a reason and why should I get in the way? I need to think about this a bit more and get my head straight. I always thought you were supposed to do the "right thing". But I guess "right for whom" is the REAL question.

27th August 8:19am

NOT feeling paranoid this morning but FEAR is lurking when it comes to sitting in the dining room. I'm not a total coward – I sat in there for tea and toast last night for about a whole sodding HOUR. I realise that the only thing I have to fear are my THOUGHTS. You know the saying "sticks and stones may break my bones but words (thoughts) will never hurt me"? What a load of bollocks! True, thoughts can't harm you physically – unless they drive you into physical danger – but they bend and warp what is going on in your head and alter how you perceive things. THAT can really hurt.

On the advice of the staff I'm building up gradually – I'm phoning Mitch and my family again and making regular contact. Give me a little time and I'll deal with the whole dining room issue. I HATE being scared of things and I generally face them and cope so I have no doubts that in a couple of days – all things being good – I'll be in there eating my meals and swinging from the metaphorical chandeliers.

12:15pm

Went for a champion walk this morning – no paranoia, no suicidal thoughts (although I was faced with a HUGE purchasing dilemma – saw a pair of REALLY COOL leather boots that I DON'T NEED and can't even BEGIN to justify... but they were CALLING to me – and not in a hallucinatory way!) So, I'm feeling pretty normal ("normal" being a relative term) and I'm quite HAPPY – gasp! I used the "H" word – and relaxed. I'm missing lunch 'cos I feel a teeny bit pukey – probably due to the meds increase but it's fine and I'm A-OK.

How many psychiatric nurses does it take to change a light bulb? One. But only if it REALLY wants to change. Ahem. See? I'm feeling well enough to make crap jokes...bummer, eh?

7:24pm

How is it possible that even with my headphones on, I can hear people bitching about me and laughing and calling me names? I feel like SHIT right now and I know EXACTLY what the trigger was: Mitch and I talked (in the third person) about suicide and dangerously explored ideas of how to kill yourself in the dorm. This was not territory I was AT ALL comfortable with and I should have nipped it in the bud. But I didn't. And now, with the help of a PRN I'm having to deal with the thoughts, feelings, and beliefs that have arisen as a consequence. God, I can be DUMB at times. This is NOT the way to end a good day. How do I feel? Paranoid, shaky and just generally scared and freaked out. I HAVE to get off the Ward or I'll start crumbling from the inside out. I NEED to be on my own and if 15mins is all I get I'll grab it with every part of me.

8:06pm

No respite. The shadowy crap in my head hitched a ride and giggled malevolently at me in a sickening haze all round my walk. Y'know, sometimes I think it would be easier not to fight, be consumed by it and lose insight. Pretty crazy, eh? But at least if I had no insight I wouldn't have the TORMENT of being aware that I'm losing it and the continual battle to keep a grip would slip gently and quietly away. Sure, I would still be paranoid but NOT paranoid AND fighting it which is pretty exhausting.

I think the pills ARE helping 'cos I feel a bit more relaxed and at ease but I'm still TERRIFIED that everyone has it in for me and is saying the most TERRIBLE things about me...and worse, making out like they all want to help me when they're really thinking shit about me. Fuck this. Fuck insight too for that matter.

8:20pm

It's amazing — WITHOUT the help of a PRN I've started feeling better over the past five minutes! I can feel the paranoia backing off and a fresh breeze has blown the dirt off my aching bones. I still feel a bit anxious but that's okay, in fact pretty much everything's okay.

28th August 7:44pm

Had a lovely (and mercifully PRN – less) Indian curry with Mitch this evening which was bloody marvellous except when we told the waitress it was our anniversary and she replied with the gem that it was the first anniversary of her uncle's death (a motorcycle accident apparently). Now, how do you respond to THAT? "Chicken korma with Nan bread?" somehow felt a little inappropriate!

I feel fine right now which is AMAZING when you consider the quantity of onion rings/curry/Nan/tablecloth that I consumed earlier. If I'm sick later feel free to have NO SYMPATHY WHATSOEVER. So. Things are cool. LONG MAY IT CONTINUE...

29th August...

30th August 7:45am

Had a decent night last night although I was somewhat jarringly awoken by a room mate of mine who shall remain nameless – Ok, it was Miriam. She woke me at 4:15 cutting about the room in her slippers, showering, getting dressed and then going back and forth for WHATEVER REASON. LOVELY. I shouldn't complain as she's doing that sort of thing much less often nowadays* and she picked a night when everyone else was on pass.

Mentally I feel fine this morning which is very cool but I'm going to be careful as today is a bit of a sad day as it is the day that Mitch and I were supposed to be getting married so I'll need to do 2 things 1. Keep things in perspective 2. Make sure Mitch is okay.

*could I tempt fate more?!

5:45pm

BAD THOUGHTS circumnavigate my skull carelessly dragging their filthy talons over the surface of my brain. They RIP and TEAR and it HURTS more than I ever thought I could. I feel and believe I am a TRULY terrible person. Fucking SCUM. Utter SHIT. And I don't feel AT ALL comfortable in my skin right now. AAAAAAAAAAAAAGGGGHH!!!!

I can't get away from myself and it's driving me NUTS. The thoughts? That I am bad, bad, BAD and worth NOTHING AS A PERSON. This all kicked off because of what I said to Katy earlier (which I don't want to write down here). I hardly spoke to Jane when she visited but that was okay 'cos she had LOADS to tell me. Now I'm back on the Ward and these bastard thoughts hitched a ride and followed me back from McDonalds chuckling evilly and heckling constantly.

I JUST WANT TO SWITCH THEM OFF BECAUSE THEY ARE BOTHERING ME.

7:35pm

I've worn out my watch face from staring at it so much. I swear AT LEAST 4 hours have past since I last glanced at it but, no, my oh-so-fashionable Bench timepiece stubbornly disagrees and INSISTS that it's only been 2¼ minutes. I want. I want time to pass so that the PRN can dissolve into my bloodstream like popping candy in a sticky glass of raspberryade. I WANT TO FEEL BETTER THAN THIS. I WANT...I WANT TO WANT 'cos NOTHING feels right at the moment and I am rattling around in my body alone in a busy, populated Ward unable to connect with anyone. I WANT to be ME.

Whoever that is.
I have NO IDEA...

31st August 8:46am

I feel like I am swimming underwater and am DESPERATE to take a breath but I KNOW what will happen if I do so I MUST hold on until I reach the surface or the water will savage my lungs and kill me. That is what living with these thoughts is like. I can't afford to obey them but when I get lost in them they surround and monopolize me and I can't "breathe" them in even though that would be easier, SO MUCH easier than challenging them. I guess part of the problem is that the thoughts don't really feel out of place. I BELIEVE them. They are very absorbing which makes it difficult to do everyday things like talking and responding appropriately to others. Sometimes I believe I am a shambling mute. Sometimes I am.

11:06am

All together now — HURRAY FOR PRNs!!! I feel much better, so much so that when I smile I can actually FEEL it inside rather than the "dead" feeling I get so used to. I LOVE this, I'm the smell of freshly cut grass, the taste of ripe strawberries and the sound of your favourite song. Let me be greedy and enjoy this for a while.

2:04pm

It feels like the contents of my head are solidifying and the neuro-transmitters and synapses are totally FUCKED. It becomes harder and harder to think in any coherent, focused fashion and speaking becomes an obstacle that is difficult to overcome.

And then there are the ghosts. The spooks that emerge from the deepest, darkest corners that torment me with noise and threats that MAY be empty — but so am I right now. I can do without this crap. I don't want a PRN.

I just want this to NEVER HAPPEN AGAIN.

5:50pm

I think the bouncing around of my mood today is probably due to the reduction of one of my meds...either that or it's take away withdrawal — I haven't had one for TWO WHOLE DAYS! I feel pretty good right now mood-wise. Let's hope it lasts...

8:11pm

Just had some FANTASTIC honey and garlic ribs for dinner which was great and much needed as I skipped lunch and dinner today. I KNOW this is tempting fate HUGELY but I feel fine at the moment and the thoughts have backed off as much as they ever do. Hopefully I'm in for a good evening/night? It's GOT to be better than yesterday's anyway.

September

1st September 8:22am

I had a good evening yesterday and because of that I felt able to have a chat with Gary about my meds and my general progress which we both agreed could be A LOT better than it currently is. It's SO FRUSTRATING. My mood was bouncing around like a trampolinist on speed yesterday and as such I was KNACKERED last night plus it's REALLY disconcerting and generally damaging not knowing how I'll be from one hour to the next. It's a CRAP situation and I think I'm allowed to be a little fed up. But I can't afford to wallow in self pity — that's a dangerous path and one best avoided.

My plans for today are to go out for lunch with a friend at 12:00pm and then Mitch is coming to visit later. I just hope I'll be in good form for both because it feels like I have NO control here and it fucking SUCKS.

I found an 11 second piece of music that gives me the chills 'cos it actually simulates, in an audible way, how it FEELS when the thoughts start escalating in my brain and eventually swarm and take over. Lovely, I know. Seriously, it's quite good to be able to play it to people as it articulates in a way that I can't what it FEELS like for me and highlights the intimidation and this-can't-be-stopped-ness of it all.

2:15pm

Feeling whacked after my lunch out and, as a consequence, my mood has unsurprisingly dipped a bit. Which is pants. Plus for

SOME REASON Lila, another patient, is REALLY focused on me today and WON'T LEAVE ME ALONE which is doing my head in. OF COURSE I realise that she is unwell it's just difficult when she refuses to leave me alone, sits on my bed, looks in my locker and plays my guitar ALL WITH OUT MY PERMISSION. GRRR.

2:40pm

Mood is getting worse and bad thoughts are starting to peck away merrily at my brain tissue. I'm just going to stay in my room on my bed until it passes. It's safe there (as long as Lila stays away).

4:15pm

Keith let me go for a walk which was cool. Still feeling nervous of staff but a bit better than how I was feeling earlier. I think the reason I get so scared of staff is that I perceive that they have all the "power" whereas I am vulnerable and have none. Plus I don't even know most of their last names let alone anything else about them, especially Agency staff some of whom I only meet once. I KNOW I get paranoid – I have some insight but would YOU feel safe in an enclosed environment with a bloke you have never met before? Yes, I realise there are other people around but I don't feel particularly trusting of them either at the moment. I feel like everyone's STARING at me and it's PISSING ME OFF.

7:31pm

I hope I didn't offend anyone with my 4:15pm entry – that WAS NOT my intention and I'm really sorry if I did. Sigh. Maybe with the change of shifts this tangled web I've woven in my head will unravel and fade into the ether. Here's hoping.

Until I feel a bit more sure about how people feel towards me I'll just hang out in my room. I think, no, I KNOW that this whole paranoia thing was kicked off by Lila this morning. She REALLY got to me — so much so that I really had to CONTROL my temper this morning. I HATE losing my cool and she pushed me pretty hard. I value my personal space and privacy to a HUGE degree in the Ward and to have BOTH invaded almost tipped me over in the anger stakes, which kind of threw me off for the rest of the day.

That's my theory anyway.

2nd September 6:15am

Woke early because Miriam was doing her best to be very, very, VERY NOISY from about 5:00am onwards. Apparently Lila was in my room AGAIN last night which was not great — that woman sure knows how to wind people up. I REALLY wish she would just leave me alone but, in all honesty, it isn't that important in the grand scheme of things and I have my MDT to think about today which is much more pressing.

I feel okay this morning. My paranoia wore off as last night continued and, whilst I might not exactly feel refreshed this morning, my thoughts are relatively clear and healthy — as much as they tend to be at the moment anyway.

5:25pm

For some reason up until 10 mins ago I was certain Caitlin and Pam had it in for me and were doing 2 things: saying terrible things about me to all and sundry and 2. plotting my transfer to some HORRENDOUS facility somewhere. I feel a little more attached to what I'm hoping is REALLY reality after finally summoning up the guts to speak to Pam. I'm just hoping that the PRN kicks in soon and does its job because this craziness is still charging around my head at warp speed and I feel all at sea and messed up.

6:56pm

Feeling better but everything feels a bit surreal right now and it's as though I'm quite separate from things – people mainly.

3rd September 8:46am

I guess I'm feeling paranoid this morning (and fragile and anxious and stressed) because I feel very wary of the staff and I'm pretty certain they're all against me. Caitlin suggested that I go to Dumbarton Hospital on my own and probably, on MOST days, I could manage in a taxi. But today? Today FEAR is ripping through me like a tornado and I'm nervous and suspicious of EVERYONE. Why would Caitlin suggest this TODAY? Because they can't be bothered with me anymore? I think that I am, on a busy Wednesday, a royal pain in the ass. I'm sorry about that. I'm wondering if my period id due because I'm really feeling freaked out and frightened, so PLEASE don't mess with my head right now.

I feel miserable and pressured already and I can FEEL that noose around my neck again... and it makes it so hard to swallow.

5:24pm

Took a PRN and caught a lift to Dumbarton with Ann, which was VERY fortuitous and cool. I felt MUCH improved after the PRN and had a good chat with Dr Fallowfield about learning to recognise coping strategies eg. NOT going for a walk when having suicidal thoughts, going and ASKING for a PRN which seem GLARINGLY obvious in the cold and RATIONAL light of day but dances and skips teasingly outwith my reach when I am ill. I think I find it difficult to request PRNs for 4 reasons 1. I totally FORGET about them 2. I think I won't be believed and so get turned away (this has never happened) 3. I feel what is happening is all my fault anyway 4. When it gets really bad I just seem to get lost in what I am experiencing and it's so tangible that I don't believe that ANYTHING could alter the status quo.

Dr Fallowfield and I are still working on ways to fix this and we talk about breathing and grounding — trying to reconnect with reality a bit and so regain some rational perspective. But it's like when I feel paranoid and/or suicidal it's as though my brain is full to bursting with negativity so much that there just isn't ANY room for solutions and positivity. I need to learn to fight HARDER, I guess.

My pass went well — just ate pizza and fell asleep with Mitch — a pretty cool afternoon really.

4th September 8:43pm

Last night was fine for me, more or less, but I was really worried about Katy who looked AWFUL and had to go home. Hope she's okay.

Lila, the human boomerang, continues to DO MY HEAD IN. She has absolutely NO respect for my privacy whatsoever. I'm not going to lose my temper over this, frankly it's not worth it, but it's tough keeping a lid on things at times especially late at night (midnight-ish) when I'm tired and she is INTRUDING. Privacy is something that is a precious, scarce commodity here and, on the whole everyone goes out of their way to respect everyone else's, so I DON'T appreciate mine being continually violated.

Mood and psychosis wise I was fine last night AND this morning which is great!

12:15pm

Not sure what to do. Dr Fallowfield and I discussed positive approaches to tackling negative mood states and I'm trying REALLY hard to implement them RIGHT now because my head is currently being compressed by a LARGE VICE and bad thoughts and suspicions are queuing up to join the party. I don't feel AT ALL good but I don't think it's at it's peak yet and I don't know whether to take a PRN or not. I kind of want to go for a walk but...AAAARRRGGHH I'm getting LOST in this.

5:05pm

One PRN, a sleep and a walk with Gary later and I feel MUCH improved.

I feel kind of nervous but excited about my new book, "The Snow Globe Journals" (shameless plug) coming out which, I think, is a big improvement on the ambivalence and negativity I felt only a few weeks ago. A sign that I'm getting better? I hope so.

7:51pm

Okay, so it does my head in when Lila comes into my room and stares RELENTLESSLY at me and refuses to leave BUT it REALLY pisses me off when she goes in AND plays my guitar WHEN I'M NOT EVEN THERE! I'm getting REALLY SICK of this and the most frustrating thing is that she doesn't seem to LEARN. GGRRRRRRRRRRRR!!!!!!!!!

5th September 7:55am

Feeling all right this morning. I had a good sleep from about 11:30pm-6:00am which was good. Went for my morning walk where again the urge to step out in front of a car/bus was pretty compelling but I was pleased that I found if I used Kim's advice to talk to myself out loud and TELL myself not to do it I could handle things well. Okay, so this technique may make me look a bit odd but, hey, if it works...?

11:39am

Michel's Mum is having an endoscopy in the hospital this morning as she is continuing to deteriorate health wise. Hoping I'll be allowed to go along and visit her...

3:14pm

Got permission to go to the endoscopy suit which was a good thing because Mitch seemed really glad to see me. As to the results nothing conclusive was found but she has to go for a CT scan so we'll see what news that brings.

4:56pm

I can feel bad thoughts rolling in like bowling balls in a ten pin alley so I'm off to distract myself in whatever healthy way I can think of. It's like the walls are bleeding black sticky oil and its got on the floor and onto my shoes and now it's creeping up my legs freezing my blood and infecting my skin. I can't seem to stop it. I TRY but it's smarter and more determined than me. Besides, I've only had 18 years experience at fighting it and it's been around waiting for me FOREVER.

6:01pm

I think that Gary was getting at me when he was talking about young people having "no direction"*. I'm trying to have direction but right now circumstances have left me with no momentum or velocity to generate a direction and give it meaning. I'm frightened right now — of what I'm thinking and how I feel. I don't want a PRN — that just validates that I'm broken. I just want EVERYTHING to GO AWAY AND NEVER COME BACK. I feel scared of the staff and it feels as though my heart wants to escape my body in a flurry of convulsions whenever I am in the vicinity of one of them. How I HATE this!!! I'm trying to make it to 7:00pm so I can order, and focus on, my take away but right now I don't feel too hungry or focused so I don't know.

I don't know.
Anything.

*Gary came and found me later and assured me he wasn't referring to me at all.

6th September 7:46am

I don't know what to write this morning. Nothing really sums this up.

6:05pm

Feeling better. My pass fell into 2 parts: before PRN/ after PRN. Before PRN I felt horribly disconnected and as though my thoughts were unravelling faster than I could put them together. It was distracting and very uncomfortable plus I felt pretty weird and out of it. It was as though someone had nicked the remote control and was channel surfing whilst I was trying to concentrate and make sense of the programmes. I couldn't put anything together properly and my brain was overloaded and fried.

One PRN later and I felt much improved. Suddenly I had the remote again and I could watch what I wanted AND control the VOLUME and BRIGHTNESS. The best thing about my pass? Seeing my cat, Casey, again!

7:20pm

Lila is doing my head in BIG TIME. SHE KEEPS COMING INTO MY ROOM although she's wily enough to sit with a very shy, quiet roommate of mine but she STARES at me constantly and her presence drives me up the wall. As such I feel unable to play my guitar, use my phone or generally relax in MY space. She is so intrusive but I feel that I can't leave either as she has the habit of poking around my stuff or helping herself to my guitar when I'm not about. The only solution I have is to keep my guitar in the office where neither of us can play it and continually get members of staff as soon as she is physically NEAR me in the room. I'm getting angrier and ANGRIER about this.

7th September 7:21am

Asked Clive if I could move rooms last night as this whole Lila situation is really DOING MY HEAD IN. If I had a single room at least if she so much as stepped over the threshold or stared through the window I would be much more confident about getting a member of staff to remove her. Basically I would have much more control over my space and hopefully

That would remove some of the ANGER and frustration that I feel. This whole issue is bringing up aspects of my personality that I am not comfortable with i.e. rage and tearfulness. I really hope that this can be sorted before I snap. This isn't blackmail it's just the way things are right now and I feel as though I am being rammed up against a wall with my face scraping against the bricks. I don't normally let people get to me and I haven't lost my temper for 16 years but I can feel badness brewing and it isn't good for anyone.

9:54am

Anger/self hatred/bad thoughts...not exactly rocket science is it? Struggling a bit with black, morbid thoughts and no doubt my early period is adding to the mix. Playing my guitar in the group room helped a bit but now the thoughts swamp me like badly fitting, itchy clothes and they're demanding my full attention. I'm tired and tired and tired of everything.

1:24pm

AAAAAAAAARRRGGGHHH!!!!!!!! Will everyone get the Hell out of my room and give me some SPACE! Jesus, I feel like a powder keg full of bad intentions and ready to blow. There's only so many walks I can go on. I feel as though I am cracking up. REALLY. And it's not going to be pretty. This is supposed to be my place of respite and free from pressure. Not right now it isn't. Obviously I am pushing for a single room. In all my admissions I have NEVER requested a room change but I think I'm justified in my reasons for the moment. For me control over my surroundings is vital and I feel I am losing my grip on that at the moment. I'm desperate to spend some time ON MY OWN just chilling out in my own space. I'm not well enough to go home yet so I NEED to find that space on the Ward. I'm fraying like an old rope and, as such, getting more and more vulnerable to breaking.

On top of all this crap I'm having a horrible day and I seriously considered throwing myself out of my Mum's car on the way to ASDA. The blurred tarmac looked inviting out of the window and the thought that I could finally "stop" lodged itself in my brain and began a noisy dance.

And then there was the cat we saw being run over. I saw TOO MUCH of the cat. That was enough.

2:50pm

THANK YOU LISA!!!! Caitlin asked Lisa if she would be willing to switch rooms with me and she said "Yes"! Hurray! I'm still feeling quite shitty but at least I'm feeling shitty in my own space without PEOPLE around me ALL THE TIME. Now I can relax. And breathe.

8th September 8:16am

Confusion. And depersonalisation. That's what was going on in my head last night. By the time night time meds came around I was so brain fried and tired that I decided to hit the hay at 10:15pm AND SLEPT THROUGH UNTIL 7:00am! Which is the best sleep I've had since the very beginning of January. THANK YOU for moving me to a single room! Feel okay this morning — got a bit of a buzzing in my head but other than that I'm fine.

1:35pm

Feel kind of out of it right now. Hmmm. I'm finding it hard to follow conversations if more than me and one other person is involved. It's like my body is present but my brain is in a whole other room. The buzzing has stopped though which is good. I'm going to Clydebank with Mum to see if that helps, failing that I am tempted to SMACK my head off something hard to see if I can get things back in place.

My resting pulse has dropped by 20 bpm since my move into a single room.

5:02pm

Worried that the staff are talking about me in the office. And not saying very nice things at that. Especially nervous of Caitlin and Alice, not sure why. I'm 60% sure I'm paranoid but that other 40% is pushing me hard. Lila has left me alone today which is good (so far...). I'm really tired after my Clydebank visit and that's probably why I am a bit...I dunno really.

6:44pm

Mitch has just left and promised me that he likes the new trainers that I bought him. He is now officially a funky dude.

Unfortunately, spent most of the evening visit distracted and worried that "people" are coming to "get me" and that I'm being spied on. Don't know whether to keep my door open — so I can see who it is — or closed — so they can't see me. Should I ask for a PRN? That means approaching staff which is a problem. I DON'T KNOW WHAT TO DO!!!! THIS IS DOING MY HEAD IN!!!

8:14pm

Feeling better. FINALLY approached a member of staff and after we talked I was given a PRN. WHY do I torture myself by waiting SO LONG to take/ask for one???

9th September 11:32am

I had a good evening yesterday and slept like a sleepy thing. I'm MUCH preferring my single room and, I think, reaping the benefit as I am feeling more relaxed and less stressed out plus I think Lila has finally taken the hint and is leaving me alone.

My MDT went well this morning and was a very chilled affair — I was so laid back you could have used me as a shelf! Dr Smith is great and really listens, which is superb, and makes an effort to put me at my ease (which is not an easy job as I get pretty nervous before MDTs). The long and not so long of it is that I get an overnight pass on Fri/Sat which I'm looking forward to — I think it's the right time.

Obviously, as I said to Dr Smith, I want everything to be PERFECT. She smiled. Ok, I said, at least I want things to be better than they are right now. She agreed and explained how she might be changing my meds again in the near future.

3:16pm

Spoke to Dr Fallowfield about "specialness" which he feels could be related to the motivation behind my high achievements and how that could have impacted on what makes me "ME". Not a lot of resolution today then but plenty to chew on for next week.

6:14pm

Feeling rubbish.

8:23pm

I don't know what to think. Or maybe I just don't WANT to think. I'm TIRED and bad thoughts are hounding me like jackals after an easy feed.

If I'm honest I think privately I'm a bit nervous of my overnight pass on Fri/Sat. I KNOW it's a bridge I have to cross and Dr Smith and the staff wouldn't be even CONSIDERING it for me if they didn't think I was ready. I just worry HUGELY about getting bad thoughts away from the safety of the Ward. This is a new road I'm walking down and at the moment I feel as though I am walking it with no shoes on.

So, just want to turn off my brain and escape for a while. Exactly how I manage that I have NO Idea...

10th September 7:28am

I felt like leaving the Ward with bad intentions last night for the first time in AGES. I think it's because I was being SWAMPED with a variety of bad thoughts — guilt, paranoia, self hate, confusion plus on top of all that I was just TIRED of pushing horrible thoughts away — I had been doing THAT ALL DAY.

11:44am

Damn. I was about 50cm away from being knocked down by a car this morning. Must TRY and be more vigilant and self aware when crossing the road. Sometimes I just can't be bothered looking left and right.

Tai Chi was good — managed 40mins this time — and went for a coffee afterwards with Charlie (the other O.T.) which was really nice. I'm feeling Okay — a bit tired but fine.

Actually there MAY be something wrong with me... Well, not WRONG exactly, but different. I've just taken a departure from my usual "Grim As Fuck" song writing style and composed a LOVE SONG for Mitch. Oh my God. I'll be turning into Celine Dion soon!!!

2:44pm

I am getting more and MORE preoccupied with things in my head and the harder I push them away the stronger they seem to push back. I'm trying SO HARD to run away from myself right now and I'm keeping as physically active as possible. But the thoughts, like the weather, are REALLY SHIT and if I'm honest? I'm scared of them. I'm scared of the way they make me feel and I'm scared of the mental avenue I'm being pushed down. I realise that I am in control here, I just wish I could get all of this crap out of my head so that I could have a bit of peace.

I feel as though my body is void of organs and the space has been filled with an oily, black, STINKING liquid and if I cut myself, black would pour out. On the surface everything looks normal and I can laugh and even make crappy jokes but I am struggling inside and this is pretty tough going.

3:15pm
Feeling pretty bad right now.
Can't really cope with other people.
Can't really cope with myself.

7:07pm
One PRN later and I feel a bit better as though someone has washed the windows inside my head and I can "see" again. But. There is still dirt smeared around the edges and I just KNOW that it will spread again. Until that happens I HAVE to keep my focus and EAT something — I can't keep skipping meals. Distraction is the order of the day so I intend to write a new song, eat a burger, have a shower, phone Mitch and listen to my MP3 player.

Here's hoping...

11th September 7:48am
Just back from my walk which was a miserable affair. God, I feel rotten this morning and I just wish I hadn't woken up. I don't know whether to ask for a PRN. I just don't know. I feel as though what I need is a hammer to crack my head open and release all of the

crap and blackness that resides there right now. I read this and think that I am shit, awful and a right moaner. I don't like myself very much at the moment and those thoughts are somehow multiplying all by themselves. I don't want to phone Mitch (or Mum) and lay all of this on them. They don't need that. I just want to stop having BAD thoughts prowling around my brain and be able to envisage some kind of future that has a positive outcome. Not like now. I'm scared of people and of the fact that I feel so DEAD inside.

Got to give myself a kick up the arse and go to breakfast, or have a cup of tea anyway.

10:21am

I CAN'T SEE how I am going to make it. These thoughts are awful and they insert terrible, visual ideas in my head about ways in which I could kill myself. They cause me to look at objects in a new suicidal light — a seemingly harmless plastic spoon stolen from the dining room opens a world of deadly possibilities until, after ½hr, I finally crack and yes, with a bit of reluctance, hand it in to Caitlin. I HATE THIS and the confusion rips my brain apart. I'm TRYING SO HARD to survive this — I'm constantly trying to suss out the right route through these thoughts and I'm terrified that I'll get it wrong. There are no second chances here. Sometimes killing myself really does seem like the right idea but so far I've managed to delay and desperately search for a different perspective to avoid it.

I'm still here.
It's just SO hard, that's all.

10:46am

AT LAST I'm getting a bit of respite from the thoughts. It's so weird and unexpected but VERY WELCOME. I can actually relax a little and not have to be so hyper – vigilant about what's going on in my head. I feel like I'm cruising down a slight slope on a road and while I still have to be careful about steering and keeping my balance I don't have to pedal as hard.

12:52pm

Sometimes I feel like I'm a ghost, that I'm not real and that I'm completely transparent. There is no substance to me and it would be easier for me just to disappear. Mum's offered to take me out to lunch to Luss but I'm nervous of the car and of leaving the Ward. So maybe not. I just don't know. I feel...unpredictable just now. I have NO idea whether I am being held together by the PRN I took earlier or whether it's worn off and this fragility I'm feeling is worryingly genuine.

I need a chat with Pam.

4:23pm

WWWWWHHHHYYYYY???????? WHY did I feel like CRAP the minute I stepped out of the front door and IMMEDIATELY all the HORRIBLE thoughts pounce on me as though they've been hanging out WAITING? I really HATE MYSELF at times. Just so you know I'm feeling ROTTEN and EDGY and VULNERABLE AND PARANOID because someone from a newspaper has just called on my mobile (how did they get my number???) wanting me to write a piece on fucking SUICIDE. Obviously I turned them down but I feel as though my safety zone has been intruded on. STAY AWAY!!!!!!!!!!!!!!!!!!!!!!!!!!!!!!

7:45pm

PRN and chat with Pam both calmed me down and as a consequence I'm feeling much less paranoid and stalked. Anger and general pissed off — ness still pour through my veins though. Because of that phone call I felt intruded on and fucked off to the max. An article on suicide?!! I feel that perhaps NOW IS NOT THE RIGHT TIME.

Not even a little bit.
No way.

12th September 9:07am

Still feeling irritated by the intrusion of that phone call yesterday but I'm trying my level best not to dwell on it too much. Besides, I have an overnight pass to look forward to and, more than anything, I want it to go really well. Mitch and I are planning to go out for a meal tonight which should be cool and as for the rest of the time? I'll just play it by ear. I'm feeling good this morning though and I feel that I'm handling things pretty well and keeping my head together. All I ask is no nasty surprises please!

8:28pm

Went out for a meal with Mitch but couldn't eat much or make much of a job of conversation because I was freaking out a bit and feeling pretty scared of everyone in the restaurant. Walking home through the town wasn't the most pleasant experience I have ever had. At all. Took a PRN at 6:30pm but it hasn't helped that much and now I'm worried that the house is going to be broken into and we'll be attacked. As such I'm nervous about going to sleep. I KNOW this is irrational but that in itself doesn't make the FEAR go away. I phoned Clive at the Ward who gave me some reassurance. I really DON'T want to go back early from my pass so I'm determined to stay put. I HATE feeling like this but I must keep moving forward.

It's HARD though.

13th September 10:50am

In the end I slept pretty well last night and it was LOVELY to wake up next to Mitch! Feeling a bit pukey and, rather worryingly, my pee was ORANGE this morning which is never a good thing. I swear to God, if my liver is playing up again I'll...GRRRRR!

Anyway, mentally I feel much better and I think that, all in all, I'm coping well.

3:30pm

Got back to the Ward about 30mins ago and to my IMMENSE relief my pee is back to a normal yellowy colour. My guess is that my liver wasn't overly thrilled with the mussels I had last night (maybe a touch ambitious!). Seriously, I felt kind of sick this morning so it probably was the mussels. Obviously I'm not going to RUSH out and order them again!!!

Anyway, mentally I'm feeling as fine as I ever do which is great. I think that, barring a few hours last night, things went well and were mercifully uneventful. I think taking the PRN and chatting to Clive helped a lot — but let's face it, I've been in hospital for 5 months so to go home and spend a night there was always going to be a bit strange. But I coped, as did Mitch, and we both rate it as a (nervous) SUCCESS.

14th September 7:28am

I'm feeling REALLY apprehensive about approaching the staff this morning probably due to the HORRIBLE dream I had last night in which they were trying to convince me that I was about to die. In it there was a mega storm going on and Caitlin took me for a walk in it. She then started freaking out and screaming "You're going to DIE!" Over and over. Not nice really.

7:48am

Went for my walk. Thought about hanging myself. Didn't. Came back. That dream is haunting me and it's hard to differentiate between daytime thoughts and feelings and 'nightmare' ones. This isn't anything new, I ALWAYS struggle getting my head together after a really visual and realistic bad dream. It FEELS real to me and I feel miserable because of it. I get confused and preoccupied and it SUCKS. I also suffer from flashbacks into it which only last a few seconds but bother me a lot and serve to disrupt my understanding and grasp of what is really going on.

10:05am

The staff are spying on me. That's what the BIG thought spinning around in my head says. I KNOW it's paranoia but let's face it — they have the keys/I don't, they have the power e.g. imposing constants etc/I am at their mercy, I don't even know most of their second names let alone any personal details about them/ they know EVERYTHING about me. And you wonder why

I get paranoid?! All I know for sure is that this feeling is too large and slippery to get hold of. I want it to leave. Or at least let me fold it up, stick it in a box and move it to a dark well hidden corner of my brain. EVERY time someone walks past my door I feel myself panicking and it's NOT GOOD. I HATE this. Shit. I'm still pretty damn sure that certain people here are thinking, if not saying, AWFUL things about me. If I was braver I would approach them and face them. Right now I'm not that courageous.

Give me a little time.
Please.

11:40am

Spoke to Caitlin. Okay, she approached me but I'm glad she did as talking to her helped dissipate the horrible, threatening fog in my head a little. She gave me a PRN and I think it's starting to work as I feel a bit more relaxed and my thoughts are like a giant knot that's gently being unravelled and put in some kind of rational order. Things are still a bit hazy and although I feel better about things I intend to be careful in the same way that you wouldn't run 800m after just having a cast removed from your leg. My plans are to go to ASDA with Mum and Mitch at 2:00pm, then work on my new song "Anxious, Restless" for the rest of the afternoon and then just CHILL.

4:02pm

I'm feeling as anxious as anything. Why? Because I CAN'T SEE A WAY OUT OF THIS. My time out was crap because this metaphorically MASSIVE BOULDER that represents my suicidal thoughts casually rolled up and stopped at my feet. It's

154

too big to either push out of the way or walk round and I don't know what to do. I think that BAD THINGS are going to happen to me sooner or later and it scares the shit out of me. It's like one of those old mechanical shoe size measuring machines crushing me from all sides. I NEED HELP with this one 'cos I don't know what I'm doing. And I'm fucking SCARED. I don't need anymore PRNs I need plans and tactics that WORK.

6:52pm
AAAAAAAAAARRRRRRRRRGGGGGGGHHHH!!!!!! Paranoia and thoughts that the staff are talking about me (IN CODE — THEY'RE CLEVER) are bouncing around my brain again. I'm so TIRED of this crap. I wish I could just SCREAM to release some of the fear and frustration I feel. Paranoia messes with my brain and laughs at me — **HAH HAH HAH FUCKING HAH!** Talking to Lydia has helped a bit but I'm still edgy and it's ONLY 7:00pm. Why does this happen? WHY??????????

15th September 7:40am
Suicidal thoughts are PULVERISING my thoughts this morning. I just can't see any other options. At all. So I went to go for my walk but as I approached the door I began retching and shaking so badly that I couldn't even make it out of the door nevermind anything else. So I chickened out and stayed on the Ward. I'm still feeling as though the staff are spying on me which sucks. I just wish I could go to sleep again and shut all of this mess out. I'm trying to convince myself that I can BEAT this but somehow I just can't see how at the moment.

8:15am

It's weird. I'm seeing peoples with fresh eyes because I never expected to see them again (I know that sounds a little dramatic but it's true) — I had mentally said my goodbyes this morning as I walked through the Ward to the exit but now it's as though my metaphorical flight has been cancelled and I've been allowed to stay for a while longer. I think I want that too. Just had my meds and PRNs so hopefully I will start feeling better about myself and the shakes and suspicions will subside. Ann is coming to take me out for a coffee at 11:00am and Leah is visiting this afternoon so I have plenty of things to look forward to. I've GOT to concentrate on positive things or else I'll find myself at that front door again and I'm still frightened that next time I'll step out into the rain and be lost forever.

9:50am

YES!!! I feel LOTS better and my head is clear for the first time in 2 days. The boulder is STILL there but it seems more distant and somehow less threatening and as such the fear and immediacy of the danger it poses is at a level I can cope with. The BEST thing though is that I can RELAX a bit and even smile and make some lame ass jokes (I use the term "jokes" loosely). It is as though the screaming in my head has finally backed off and my thoughts have careered from negative and frankly NOT making a huge amount of sense to calmer and more coherent. Thank God for that. Oh yes.

2:08pm

Had a great chat with Ann which was lovely — she's a star and a sparkly one at that. Just awoken from an hours nap — don't know why I'm so TIRED at the moment — probably due to PRNs and too much of that darn thinking business. I can't afford to waste energy thinking about "bad stuff"

Seriously, OBVIOUSLY I don't bring the bad thoughts on, it's as though they jump all over me from nowhere and I've got to find a way to shift them without becoming preoccupied and absorbed by them. Which is kind of like trying to juggle fog. Pretty damn difficult. Maybe taking PRNs early IS the answer — it certainly worked today. I guess if I knew the answer to that I wouldn't be here I'd be in my diamond castle greedily counting my gold and silver pieces! Must continue to stay alert and cut off any bad thoughts before they become a problem.

Which is tiring.

4:39pm

It was lovely seeing Leah but now that she's left I've suddenly realised how KNACKERED I am. Must stay focused and push that boulder away 'cos it's rumbling forward again and I...CAN'T... GET...AROUND...IT. It's tough 'cos I'm feeling a bit paranoid about Leah and I'm a bit freaked out generally. It makes me...it just makes me think bad things about myself and the solutions that I am coming up with are horrible and not healthy. It feels like the gears in my brain have jammed and I'm having difficulty shifting from the mindset I find myself locked into to. I'm NOT quitting yet though. I'm bloody well going to finish "Anxious Restless" and then take a shower. I'd like to go for a walk but it's pissing down and anyway I' don't know if that's such a cracking idea right now.

7:50pm

I'm pretty shaky and anxious right now although thankfully the suicidal thoughts I was having have faded out in the last 15 minutes which is a relief. I'm going to have a chat with Una about the electric shock sensation I'm getting on my arms and to see if she can help me undo the vicious knot in my stomach so I can face actually eating something of substance.

16th September 8:32am

Why the Hell do I have to wake up when all I want to do is continue on in black oblivion? God, it's a STRUGGLE this morning and bad thoughts and paranoia are chasing me HARD. It's so difficult to push them away as they're like a continually dividing cell multiplying and multiplying and multiplying. I'm so fed up of feeling like this – it needs to STOP. I'm so TIRED of being here mentally and physically and the thoughts are just as insistent as ever. This sucks. It would be SO MUCH EASIER to just QUIT and stop fighting this but I'm trying REALLY HARD to take others' feelings into consideration but, you know, in a way I'm kind of PISSED OFF with them for that. I feel blackmailed and manipulated. And angry.

I know.
I know I am a terrible person.

12:14pm

Feeling a bit better due to chat with nurse, sleep and PRN. Still feeling pretty depressed though and I guess a bit paranoid but not as bad as earlier.

MDT went fine and I'm having a second mood stabiliser reintroduced so fingers crossed that should help. Passes are being decided on later in the week.

Still 70% sure that people are talking about me (nastily) and judging me. The other 30%? It's a constant battle to decide which is right...

7:10pm

FUCK! Mitch has just left after telling me that I'm being paranoid because I'm worried about encountering the night staff nurses, who I THINK are Katy and Clive. Why am I worried? I'm really not all that sure but basically I think that the handover report from one shift to the next will be full of bad stuff about me and as such they'll have it in for me which makes me feel nervous and scared of them. I KNOW (and agree with Mitch) that this is paranoia but that doesn't stop me being scared and feeling as though my stomach is in a GIANT knot. Right. I WILL approach the staff immediately after the report and try and knock this fucker on the head. Then maybe I'll be able to EAT something...

I think the reason I get so freaked out about changes of shifts is that I've just got my head around one group of people when KERBLAM a whole new team come on shift and I have NO IDEA what they know or think about me. This bothers me and paranoia lurks in the wings. I'm an easy target.

8:40pm

I'm playing that waiting game — only it's not a game and no one is playing. It's called "Waiting for the PRN to work" and it better bloody well work FAST cos I'm feeling worse by the minute. I'm a swimmer with lead weights attached to her legs and arms gradually being sapped of strength and pulled under. I'm tired and this is SO HARD because part of me really doesn't want any of this life anymore. Depression sucks the blood from your veins and the marrow from your bones and it rapes and pillages your feelings of self worth and desire to live. I HATE being this person and I wish to GOD I could change. Work PRN. Work, please.

I spoke with Katy and felt a bit less paranoid about her but the suicidal thoughts are like a tsunami building in my head and I DON'T KNOW how to push it back or get out of the way.

17th September...

18th September 7:43am

This depression hounds me like a pack of angry dogs full of steel teeth and murderous intent. They are quick and eager and oh so attentive to their task. Which is? Twofold: making me feel like shit and persuading me that suicide IS the only option if I want to get out of this. I need to stand firm but the ground beneath me is marshy and doubtful and these fucking dogs are SO persistent — I fight one off and another takes its place. They can afford to rest and regain their strength when another one is savaging me. I can't. I KNOW this sounds like a "poor little me" story but I'm at a loss as to how else to describe how I'm feeling.

I missed out on my walk this morning because there are more, many more larger dogs waiting patiently for me outside and I

NEED to be sensible and not take risks. At least not STUPID ones anyway. I wish to GOD this would just GO AWAY. What is it that I have done to deserve this???

10:19am

Thought about not coming back from the dentist. Thought about lots of horrible things. But they were just thoughts. The thing is that all I have in my head are THOUGHTS and they scrape and burn and generally mess with me. Continually. I NEED to focus on other things — good things. But I'm wading through deep, murky water and I can only move slowly for fear of overbalancing into the dark, muddy depths. I HATE this. Right — distraction techniques required. I WON'T let this beat me. No way. (Y'know what? I even LIKED getting a filling because the pain reminded me that I was alive and present. Terrific.)

11:00am

I KNOW I have to be patient. I have to believe that things will get better than this. That I won't feel like I'm dead inside. When I feel like this I don't really care about myself. That is something I NEED to fix because not caring about my self leads me down many dark, convoluted alleyways all leading to places I don't much want to visit. I AM feeling A BIT better though and the sodden, dense weight that was pressing down on me earlier has lifted to some extent and I find I don't need to concentrate so hard on appearing "together". Maybe I should've taken a PRN earlier? I just felt a bit nervous of approaching the staff and asking for one. A lot nervous actually.

3:57pm

Feeling much improved which kind of follows my pattern at the moment: crap morning/good afternoon/crap evening. I have no idea as to why this is happening , I'm just hoping things will get better with the introduction of my new mood stabiliser. Right, I'm off to find Gary for a chat.

5:30pm

The Rottweilers have been let loose in my head again and, although they and their SAVAGE teeth are still distant, I can feel their presence and it panics me. I'm going to ask for a PRN to try and ward off the howling and baying depression and BAD THOUGHTS that I can feel catching in my throat. Goawaygoawaygoawaygoawaygoaway!!! Sometimes I REALLY WISH I could cry and at least release some of this torment.

7:25pm

Is my mood affected by the psychosis OR is my psychosis affected by my mood? Personally, I don't have a CLUE. I sure hope someone does. Feeling a LITTLE better from the PRN but still feel a bit rocky in my head so I need to be CAREFUL...

19th September 7:43am

I don't see the point in even ASKING to go for a walk at the moment as either one of two things will happen — 1. I won't be allowed 2. I'll start vomiting as soon as I get out of the door NOT because I'm going to try and kill myself but because of the stress and anxiety that the bad thoughts I am having are causing me. These thoughts are NOT about suicide but they are still pretty horrible hence the retching. Yet again I am nervous of the staff this morning, but hopefully that will wear off as the day continues...hopefully.

9:10am

Took a PRN about 30 minutes ago and already I'm starting to feel a bit better – which is remarkable. Maybe Gary slipped me a placebo and...SHUT UP! I've finished my song for Alicia so that's SOMETHING positive I guess and I'm off out ON MY OWN later to buy a new hooded top as it's getting a bit chillier outside. Gripping stuff, eh? Still feeling a bit nervous of the staff but not as bad as before.

11:46am

It's weird. In a good way that is. My bad thoughts and loathsome mood have evaporated somewhat and I feel a bit like...well, like ME again. I can laugh and joke and feel at ease with myself which is GREAT! Magically, I also feel less stressed by everyone and more in control. But as to how long this lasts I have NO idea – guess I'd better make that hay whilst the proverbial sun shines. I've tentatively agreed on a trip to Luss with Mum and Mitch this afternoon so I'll see how that goes. I feel a MASSIVE meringue on the horizon (purely for medical reasons, obviously!)

1:35pm

Still doing okay. Even coped with the saleswoman in the hoody shop looking at me as though I was a TOTAL IDIOT because I couldn't put the hanger back in the top that I tried on. No cool Animal hoodies in my size so I headed along to Barnardos and bought one for £2.99. EXCELLENT!

Suicidal thoughts are still lurking but they can lurk all they want just as long as it's at a level I can cope with.

Which it is.

1:52pm

Michel's Mum has terminal cancer and according to the doctor it's only a matter of weeks. The only blessing is that she spends most of her time asleep and is unaware of what is going on.

Poor Mitch, I'm REALLY worried about how he's going to handle this emotionally. He's a bit fragile at the moment and this is a HORRENDOUS situation to contend with.

Me? I feel numb and sick and all I want to do is sleep and get away from all of this for a bit. I've told Mitch to call or come over whenever he needs to. I WILL be there for him.

4:26pm

I'm certain the staff are talking about me and laughing at me in the office. I'm also pretty certain...ah never mind. I'm hoping it's all bollocks and that a PRN will fix me. The PROBLEM is that I have to approach Dorothy first and that scares the pants off me.

20th September 8:23am

Someone in my life is dying. And mean thing no.1 is that I don't really care about them to a huge extent – I'm far more worried about Mitch. Mean thing no.2 is that I don't know how I'm supposed to cope and be strong through all of this when being ME isn't where I want to be right now. This is a shitty situation for everyone involved. I wish I could just evaporate into the air and have everybody's memories of me erased so that no one would miss me. I'm so tired of feeling like this and I'm so tired generally. I'm SO tired of MOANING and knowing that paranoia and other stuff are just around the corner wearing balaclavas and they're ready to jump me. This is shit. Poor Mitch's Mum. I wouldn't wish that on anyone. I just hope to God she just falls asleep and slips away. Anything else would be awful for her. I don't want her to suffer and I don't want Mitch suffering any more than he is already.

12:49pm

I HATE THIS. I HATE EVERYTHING about it — there are NO redeeming features. At all. Let me spell it out: Mitch's Mum has been given 2 weeks. Oh my God. And how do I react? I am sure that everyone is talking about me and plotting against me (I KNOW YOU ARE). I CAN'T CHANGE THIS BIG, BAD LUMP of metal that has taken the place of my heart. I wish…I MORE than wish I was dead and I'm ANGRY that I can't do anything about that wish right now 'cos Mitch really needs me. Fucking SUPER, isn't it?

4:47pm

Just been out to buy some stamps. Picture the scene — me all anxious and paranoid to the max when this guy KICKS OFF in the newsagents because they won't accept his £50 note and he (the guy) has totally run out of fags and is FREAKING OUT. Smashing. I went and found sanctuary by the cold meat freezer and hid there until the guy left. Not exactly the best therapeutic intervention moment of my life so far.

I'm still SURE that the staff are talking about me and this magnifies at report time because they ARE talking about me only I HAVE NO IDEA what is being said. That fries my brain and the paranoia transmogrifies exponentially into panic confusion and FEAR. It's stupid and frustrating because I KNOW if I confront the person/s I'm having the problem with (and maybe ask for a PRN) I can halt it in its tracks. I KNOW THAT. But...EVERYTHING in me is telling me to hide out in my room and avoid everyone wherever possible so it's self perpetuating and brutal and nasty and insidious and all the rest of it. FUCK.

7:11pm

I CAN'T LET THIS BEAT ME. I just can't. I need to be strong/stronger/strongest for Mitch. I have NO IDEA how he's going to handle all of this. This is just the beginning – then there's the final days, the death, the funeral and coping with the aftermath. I would put my feet firmly on the ground and be a support to him – the thing is that I'm having trouble finding the ground right now and I feel all off balance.

The paranoia-fest that is the report is about to begin so I'll just stay put under my duvet and hopefully if I hide well enough, you never know, maybe fear won't find me...

21st September...

22nd September 8:51am

Mitch phoned to say he's off down to his Mum's right now as our GP is making a house call and then the MacMillan nurses are stopping by. Me? I feel fine this morning (touch wood) which is good on lots of different levels: good for me/good so that I can be strong for Mitch/good so that I'm not a distraction from his Mum. Mitch has got ENOUGH to deal with.

11:36am

STILL FEELING OKAY! Wearing my new girly, girl denim skirt which, cunningly, is long enough to hide my "Oh my God, PLEASE shave me!" legs. I'm doing all right although I might need a sleep later as one of my meds is making me knackered (could be the elephant darts).

Haven't heard back from Mitch. He said he'd call after the doc had been. I can't even say "Fingers crossed all is fine" 'cos it's not — it's just this horrendously horrible state of affairs and I feel helpless.

3:13pm

My brain has stopped. Somehow all the gears in it have JAMMED and all I know is that the staff are out to get me. All of them. I feel sick inside and little spiders of suicidal thought are crawling over my feet, up my body and are beginning the deliberate task of weaving their webs of self doubt and self hatred. I've played my guitar, gone for a walk, had a shower, watered the plants, written this sodding diary (which doesn't even get CLOSE to how I really feel). Even if I spoke to the staff I wouldn't know what to say.

Mum phoned for a chat and I went "Uh huh, yeah, no" etc when what I wanted to do was scream "LEAVE ME ALONE!!!" So I made a lame excuse and hung up. God, I'm pathetic.

7:20pm

Two people scare the pants off me today, well, three actually: Kim, Lydia and Katy. Which is dumb, futile and self defeating as part of me knows that they are ALL excellent nurses and cool people but the other side of me is TERRIFIED of them and totally freaked out. Which sucks. Big time. So. What to do? Well, I REFUSE to hide in my room — tempting as that option is — I'm going to try and have a conversation with Katy (she is my Named Nurse after all) and hopefully diffuse the general CRAPNESS I feel.

Why is hard stuff NEVER easy to do???

8:10pm

Haven't made it out of the room yet. Shit.

23rd September 6:40am

Ideally, I'd like a PRN at breakfast time to knock this STUBBORN paranoia on the head. But that all depends on who my nurse is today. Paranoia is FOUL and, regardless of any distraction techniques, continues to hammer away inside my brain. Imagine you are sure you overheard a friend say something AWFUL about you. It doesn't matter how many times you wash your hair/ play your guitar/change your clothes etc those words would still FIRE around your brain in a mental whirlwind speeding up and up and up until you go NUTS. Of course you may have misheard your friend or taken what was said out of context. Multiply by 100 and you're getting to where my head is at. It's fucking SHIT. And NOTHING I seem to do at the moment works. All suggestions welcome.

8:24am

The paranoia has backed off a bit since the 7:00am PRN which is cool especially as Kim is my nurse. 2 facts: 1. Kim is great (and owes me a tenner for saying that) 2. For God knows what reason she SCARES THE PANTS OFF ME. However, since the paranoia has diminished I have managed 2 mini conversations with her and I will continue to talk to her — no big one to ones, just a passing word in the corridor and hopefully all will be well.

12:49pm

Wow, I hate MDTs. I felt as nervous as a turkey on Xmas Eve. However, nerves aside, it seemed to go quite well. If I had been less nervous at the time (I appreciated it in retrospect) it was faintly ironic that I was discussing paranoia — particularly paranoia associated with the staff — and all the while Kim (of whom I'm just a teensy bit nervous of today) was present. I just couldn't look at her. Sorry. But all in all I held it together even though a big part of me wanted to SCREAM " DO YOU HAVE ANY IDEA HOW CRAP THIS IS???!"

1:40pm

Feeling the jangly, jarring and unpleasant rattlings of paranoia and God, do I wish it would go away. Tried to approach Kim in the office but couldn't. Quite. Manage. It. I shouldn't be surprised — I'm knackered and there's a LOT of confusion going around in my head. The fear is general right now and I feel kind of sick. I'm hoping it will sod off. Please?

4:02pm

Just left Dr Fallowfield after beginning the session feeling as spooked and freaked out as a wet cat. Feeling a bit better now but still nervous of staff. Dr Fallowfield asked me how it felt – I replied it was like millions of spiders crawling all over me and they just ain't shifting. Not nice.

5:30pm

See Dr Fallowfield sit in the office and talk to Kim for 1½ hours doesn't make me paranoid AT ALL. Really.

24th September 7:20am

I have rocks in my head this morning and they're crashing about causing me to wince and beg for paracetamol. My head hurts, my neck hurts and my eyes hurt. But apparently my capacity for moaning is still intact. Ah well, at least it's distracting me from the HORRIBLE thoughts that are careering around my brain this morning. It's hard to think coherently when your head is pounding and right now that's just fine by me.

11:54am

Walking around the local town is kind of like stepping into a freezing shower – it's nice when it stops. That's not really fair but depression permeates the air there and it DOES in a way reaffirm that things could be worse. Or maybe that's just me. Maybe.

3:36pm

Feeling crap. Mitch is having a shite time and is barely speaking and showing little or no emotion. This is HARD. For everyone. He's coming over again at 6:00pm and I don't have a CLUE what I can do to mend this other than hold his hand, tell him I love him and be there for him. If he wants to yell he can yell, if he wants to cry he can cry, if he wants to joke he can joke — I don't care. I just worry that he is suppressing everything and is in danger of falling to bits. What do I DO?

8:55pm

Mitch seemed in better spirits when he came to visit earlier and I'm doing pretty well too — okay, a few auditory hallucinations but nothing scary — just my name and footsteps when there's no one around. I try and keep my MP3 player on as much as possible and implement Dr Smith's Cognitive Behavioural Therapy (CBT) techniques e.g. rationalising and challenging the bad thoughts on paper.

Just written a new song which is a good sign...for me at least.

25th September 8:44am

I'm doing a LOT better than last night which was pretty foul later on. This morning I'm okay and looking forward to going out on pass this afternoon. I'm a little worried that Mitch will be pissed off that I don't want to go and visit his Mum but, frankly, I'm just nervous that something happens and I won't be able to cope with it. Selfish, aren't I? Yup.

On a brighter note I've died some of my hair bright blue. Why? Why the Hell not! Keith's my nurse today which is a little weird 'cos he's never been before. But that's okay. I trust him.

10:35am

Feeling paranoid again but at least I've figured out it's paranoia from the CBT sheet that all the staff are encouraging me to use. I mostly worried about Caitlin (God knows why) but I need to get my head together if my pass this afternoon is to benefit Mitch and ME. Caitlin is just freaking me out a bit and I think she has bad things planned for me. Not sure what to do about this...

12:45pm

The PRN did its stuff and as a consequence I now feel much more together and sure of how I feel about people. I also feel a lot more positive about this afternoon's pass and I'm looking forward to spending some time out with Mitch. I feel fine about the staff now which is cool.

5:02pm

Had a good relaxing time with Mitch – went for lunch, had a walk, slept from 3:00–4:30pm. He seems better than yesterday – less tense and distracted. I'm doing fine except from suffering from a side effect of one of my medications which makes me feel as though I am immersed in clay. Nasty.

7:25pm

All the negative emotions that have been swirling around in the ether have now landed on my head. Fuck. I feel depressed and scared although of what I'm not sure. I'm not paranoid about the staff though which is a GOOD THING. I have been keeping myself VERY busy since I came back but I'm knacked and I've run out of things other than watch the tumble dryer dry my top, write this and listen to music. Christ, what a COLOSSAL

MOANER I am. I guess I feel I HAVE to be strong for Mitch 'cos if I'm not strong for him he's going to cave in. It's written all over his face. The thing is that I'm not really that strong at the moment – it's more of an illusion of strength than the real McCoy. And I'm scared I can't be strong enough for both of us. What happens then?

9:50pm

I'm struggling a bit still. My cunning plan is to GO TO SLEEP EARLY. That may or may not pan out...

10:40pm

Went to find Katy to try and offload some off the crap that is creating havoc inside my head but when she asked me what was wrong all I could do was stand there in silence and stare at the linoleum. Grrrrrrr! She sent me away to WRITE DOWN was I was thinking. I'll give it a shot...

11:02pm

Wrote about the bad thoughts I was having and handed the piece of paper into Katy. Now paranoia is jumping all over me and I'm sure she gave me a placebo earlier and that she is talking about me on the phone to Caitlin RIGHT NOW to put me on constants. AAAAAAAAAARGH!

I HATE THIS!!!!!!!!!!!!!!!!!!!!!!

26th September 8:31am

Okay, so last night was pretty HORRIBLE. I was so WORRIED about so many things: Michel, getting electric shocks on my arms, things being too loud/ too bright, Michel, seeing flashes of light, bad thoughts, being put on constants, Michel, Michel's Mum, Michel, Michel...

Katy asked me to try and write down what I was thinking about with regard to the suicidal thoughts I was having (I couldn't really talk) in my own time. I couldn't do it. I tried and procrastinated but as soon as I started to get down to the nitty gritty it was as though my brain froze with an echo of "Don't tell!" reverberating around my head. I get lost inside those thoughts sometimes and it can be hard to find a way out. Sometimes medication is the only answer.

3:29pm

My pass was good — had a lovely time with Mitch: we ate lunch in the Square, went for a walk and window shopped. Then we came up to my folks' house, I had a shower and then went and lay down with Mitch which was lovely. Just spending relaxed time with him and not having to clock watch is great. The Ward makes it as easy as possible for you to have visitors and is very accommodating but nothing beats being at home (sort of). Mitch is worrying me though. Quite a lot. He's awfully quiet and grimaces when he doesn't think I'm looking at him. Hmmm.

5:30pm

Had a chat with my Dad and he managed to convince me that the rising tide of paranoia that was welling up in me was exactly that — paranoia. I'm still figuring out what to do about it. I'm at a bit of a loss. I don't like myself very much at the moment and I feel I'm not being much of a help to Mitch.

11:14pm

Felt a lot better around 7:00pm/7:30pm. Which was nice. Heh heh. Had a lovely meal at the Commodore with Mitch and then headed back to my parents' where I fell asleep in my fiancé's arms. Fantastic.

27th September 10:09am

Woke up at 9:30am ish after sleeping for AGES. Woke up with Mitch which was GREAT. Feeling a bit stressed out with regards to my wedding dress as I've put on a little weight since the last measurements were taken but hey, welcome to the wonderful world of antipsychotics! Anyway, I slept well apart from dreaming I was being spied on by stealth helicopters.

4:11pm

My 3:00pm coffee date with my friend Kayla was good on one level — we had a nice chat and she told me about her holiday to San Fran/ I gibbered about how I was doing etc. The bad thing was I felt I was being spied on and that people were listening into our conversation. I KNOW I'm paranoid but that in itself does bugger all. Plus I'm out of PRNs. Great.

Back home now chilling with Mitch so hopefully thing will improve of their own volition.

4:31pm

Mitch has just popped out before I could get the words together to tell him how I'm doing. My brain is starting to spin slowly.

5:25pm

Back at the Ward — spoke to Mitch. Still feel a big knot in my stomach and my head is pounding. Feeling a bit edgy and nervous.

7:17pm

Felt a bit better and went for a walk which was okay. Played my guitar in the group room for a while — it was cool to have some privacy and belt out some mildly out of tune songs without anyone overhearing. Now? Now I'm preoccupied with worrying about staff. I'm worried they're saying awful things about me. And thinking things. And planning things. I don't know what. Shit. Right, shower time. I KNOW I'm supposed to use distraction techniques when I think people are against me — they ARE — but how exactly they help I don't know. I feel freaked out and shaky and anxious and nervous and I'm REALLY TIRED — bring on tomorrow...

8:16pm

Okay, been for a walk to Costcutter's and got my head on a little straighter. I'm being paranoid. I feel TERRIBLE for it — like I AM an awful person but at least I recognise it for what it is. Time for a CBT sheet. The problem is I'm out of usable paper — I had a coke meets paper accident earlier on which was pretty messy.

28th September 7:01am

I had the weirdest of dreams last night 1. My legs wouldn't stop bleeding regardless of how many dressings and bandages I applied and 2. I found myself in this boarding school for domestic cleaners. I was given a blue uniform but soon realised if I put it on and followed instructions I would gradually turn into a plastic zombie like most of the 'people' who were there.

How do I feel today? Like I wish I was either the only person on the planet or that I just wasn't here. I feel OVERWHELMED by my life and I have NO IDEA what to do about it. I can't even talk about it. This will stay in my head until I find out how to eradicate it, purge it, and generally expunge it. God, I talk/write crap sometimes. But the sentiment is true nonetheless.

8:00am

I'm SO SICK of hating myself. Yes. Yes, suicidal thoughts lurk. Of course they do.

9:27am

Asleep is the safest place to be. My dreams might be scary but they're just dreams. I don't know what to do and time ticks ever MERRILY on.

12:50pm

Went for a walk with Gary which was fine. Kinda. Just had lunch and have BAD indigestion so I'm going to ask for some more Gaviscon.

7:20pm

Went for a walk with the intention of going to 'the place' NOT to do anything, just to check things out. Been feeling very nihilistic this evening so it seemed like a good idea. I was 2/3 of the way there when I heard a man laughing in a really sneering, horrible way. There was NOBODY around. NO ONE. Anyway, being a big chicken I was spooked out of my focus and before I realised it I was back at the hospital entrance. WHAT was THAT all about? I'm actually FEELING BETTER and relieved. Just "relieved" that's all; that'll do, and "better" is good as well.

29th September 9:46am

ABSOLUTELY KNACKERED. One of my meds is knocking me for six but hey, if it sorts out my head that's fine by me. Otherwise I feel okay and I'm doing fine mentally. Last night was quite funny. Dorothy had a shocker when the shelf of the medication trolley collapsed and the water jug (full) smashed on the floor. Water went EVERYWHERE. Dorothy, needless to say, was NOT happy. I reckoned she had gone "OFF HER TROLLEY"! Boom boom! Anyway, I was okay last night barring a minor episode of paranoia which I sorted with a CBT sheet and a quick word with Kim and Dorothy so that was cool.

10:42am

I was on the phone to Mum in the bathroom when I wandered out briefly, still on the phone, to find one of the nursing auxillaries holding a piece of paper and talking to one of my new room mates, Martine. INSTANTLY the thought "he's gathering information about me" fired into my brain and started pinging around in my headspace. AAAAAAARRRGGHH!!! WHY does this happen?!! Of course I challenge it, it's just it's a bit like David vs Goliath "The Sequel" and David's forgotten his sling. Grrrr. I know I should write out a CBT sheet but I also know the 'balanced' conclusion will be "I'm paranoid". So what do I DO about it? Talk to staff or PRN or both. I think I'll go and find Gary for a chat.

1:49pm

TIRED again. What a TOTAL moaner I am: for God's sake 20 weeks ago I would have taken oblivion 24hrs a day PLUS being continually branded on the soles of my feet and well, EVERYWHERE, over what I was going through mentally and now? Now all I can do is bitch and complain about comparative trivialities that continue to bug me. I'm seeking something I just can't reach, perfection. To be fair though I just REALLY want things to be at a stage where I can cope in the community again and NOT have HUGE compulsions to kill myself or get paranoid out of my face. I'm definitely climbing that ladder but my hands and feet are sore and I need to take my time. I don't want to fall.

7:25pm

Fuck. Mitch is having a HELLISH time — he's obviously really worried about his Mum, looks exhausted, is worried about me and is generally struggling. I DON'T KNOW WHAT TO DO.

No, I DON'T KNOW WHAT TO DO.

I could cry when I see him looking like this. He managed to keep up a front for about 20 minutes (I lasted 30) before this crumpled and defeated look overtook him and I had to convince him over and over that I LOVE him and that of course I WILL marry him. I don't have the luxury of being weak, at least in front of him, at the moment.

8:44pm

Kim had to put up with "weak Suzy" this evening which must have been a joy. My apologies for that. The reason I wanted to talk with her was that I had a rash idea of going for a walk and doing something stupid. Then I thought "no, I'll ask for a PRN", then I thought "just talk to them". So at least there was cognitive progress of some description, I suppose. I still feel quite shit but not suicidal and the grumbling paranoid thoughts that are MILDLY making themselves known in the background are irritating more than anything else.

30th September...

October

1st October 7:55am

I've got Kim as my nurse today which is cool.

11:40am

Alicia and Kathleen have organised a trip to Luss but unfortunately I'm not feeling too well physically (side effects) so I'd rather stay near my bed and the...er...loo.

12:01pm

I kind of felt like I was walking a very narrow window ledge this morning — on the one side — safety, security and relative peace of mind and on the other horrible thoughts, paranoia and terrible plans. I was safe on the ledge but at the same time it was a dreadful, scary place to be — anything could happen at ANY time. Anyway, I feel like I'm off the ledge and standing comfortably behind a closed window and things are a Hell of a lot better positioned than they were earlier.

Physically I'm feeling a lot better too. Tired though. Do I EVER stop moaning? Apparently not.

3:32pm

Mum came to visit out of the blue which was great but boy, was I knackered after she left! Also a bit paranoid that the more of my diary Kim reads the more she judges me>dislikes me>judges me AGAIN>can't STAND me>spreads the word to the rest of the staff and so forth and so on...but the only way I have the bottle to tell her this — cos face to face just ain't happening — is to GIVE HER MY DIARY and so the whole merry go round begins again.

This whole paranoia thing pisses me off and the FEAR that goes along with it is wearing and confusing. Late afternoons/early evenings always seem to be the worst time. From a distance it looks SO simple and clear but when you get close you can see how convoluted and messed up it is.

MOST OF ALL? Most of all I wish it would just GET LOST! Sometimes I don't know what to believe anymore and it's like my brain jams and shudders trying to figure this whole thing out and make sense of it. It's as though my gut instinct has gone AWOL. Obviously, I still know right from wrong but opinions and SUSPICIONS are much more slippery.

Actually, having written all this I feel more focused and as though I have a better handle on things.

At least I think I do!
Catharsis rules!

7:03pm

TIRED! Yawned and zzzd my way through Mitch's visit but even I was alert enough to pick up his hopes voiced for me to get a weekend pass. The thing is I JUST DON'T KNOW. I've got to be careful not to RUSH things. Being progressive is one thing — being reckless and stupid is quite another. Both Michel and I need NO backward steps just now so I will do my best to eradicate unnecessary risks and take forward steps ONLY when the road looks clear.

2nd October 7:00am

Okay, so I felt RUBBISH last night in two ways: 1. a sudden onset of depressive mood that hit home around 8:30pm (Clive let me take my night time meds early) and then by this HORRIBLE unsteady, pukey feeling that wrecked my plans of an early night (I'd hoped to get to sleep early and hide from the depression) which left me gingerly drinking water and then later, eating cereal in the dining room until I felt I could face my bed.

This morning I feel fine, and no doubt I will continue to do so until about an hour after I take my meds. I know I'm moaning 'cos I realise full well that they help and that this is just a necessary phase — it's just a nuisance, that's all.

8:05am

Ah SHIT. Conspiracy Theories against ME are racing around my head all kicked off by seeing Patrick and Kim talking intently in the office. I've seen them do this a THOUSAND times before but for some reason this morning>they're plotting to harm me. Obviously part of me is contesting this or I wouldn't be writing this entry. God, sometimes I could really do with a cigarette. STRESS! Why do I torture myself with this crap? It really sucks. And while it makes no sense it kind of DOES at the same time. Decided to go for a walk to clear my head. Which helped. Going to be doing some work on my social phobia today with Kathleen which, for SOME reason, is probably adding to my stress levels.

1:09pm

Took a PRN at around 10:50am and only started to feel even slightly better around 30 minutes ago. I don't know what to do.

Do I continue to fight this/give in/find a member of staff/go for a walk or what? Physically I feel quite rotten too — headache, nausea and TIREDNESS etc so unless today's Luss trip is just a coffee and NOT a walk I'm counting myself out.

How do I feel mentally? I feel as though I am grains of sand being sifted through a reality colander and everything is ALL OVER THE PLACE. I'm not at all certain about what I hear or even what I'm SAYING at the moment. It's cruel, insistent, persistent, scary, anxiety provoking and generally horrible. I worry about what people are saying so I put on my MP3 player on to block it out. I then worry about what I can't hear so I take it off etc etc. I usually end up with one headphone in and one off. Grrrr!

7:14pm

Paranoia is an angry, NOISY dog that yowls all day and night and won't let its owner have PEACE. My brain is knackered from all of the tortuous procrastinations and contortions that it has put itself through today. It's SUCH A WASTE of energy and time and also has the capacity to PISS ME OFF ROYALLY. I know the pattern, I know how it works but I'm damned if I've figured out a way to beat it on my own(PRNs aside)

It's still early and I'm nervous of meeting Lydia because I have NO IDEA what Kim has told her about me in the report. Not sure whether to lurk in my room or go for the head on meeting in the office.

I can tell you which is more appealing right now...

3rd October...

4th October 10:01am

Had a great night's sleep and I'm feeling okay this morning. The anti emetics seemed to have done their job and as such I feel much less sick. Ollie (my younger brother) very kindly put a whole load of cool new tunes on my MP3 player 'cos in my technophobic ineptitude I get scared that I'm going to blow up the computer. Which is probably what would happen. Probably.

12:40pm

Back at the Ward and I feel really CRAP and kinda confused at the moment as to what is real and what isn't. Hmmm. My head is buzzing and I can't make up my mind what to do about it. It's weird — I have to make an extra effort with everything I look at/hear/think to make sense of it all. I've just taken a PRN so I'm hoping that will help.

3:02pm

Mentally — okay. Physically — a bit poor. Need to rest up for a bit. Mitch and I discussed the Pass and we both reckoned it went pretty well I just need it to have a bit more definition and focus to try and stave off the bad thoughts more. Might work. Might not. Definitely worth a try though. I think I stand a fair chance of getting a 2 night pass next week (if Dr Hamilton agrees — Dr Smith is on holiday).

Holy shit! Dr Hamilton mentioned the "d word" (discharge) to me yesterday! That was a shock, a good one, but still a shock! Need to get my head around that one.

3:22pm

Just had a chat with Dr Hamilton and she suggests I go to London with Mitch on Friday. I can see where she's coming from but in all honesty I think it's a bad idea this time around. Basically neither of us can really afford for me to go to London on THIS trip, although it would be good for Mitch to have company should the inevitable — his Mum dying — happen.

5:57pm

Felt well mincey when I spoke to Pam, so much so that we agreed that a PRN was in order. So one PRN later and how do I feel. CRAP, I'm afraid. I believe that EVERYONE staff/patients /SHOs/Consultants/friends AND family are plotting against me and continually talking about me. They all HATE me. Back OFF please. WHY DON'T I FEEL BETTER??? WHAT DO I DO??? A CBT sheet won't help. Maybe. I'll try it. It can't make things worse. Felt a bit better on my walk but I can only be outside on my own for so longFORSOLONGFORSOLONGAHFUCKIT. It's like everything is being SHOUTED inside my head and shoved from one side to the other.

7:01pm

Aaaaaah. Feeling the paranoia melting away like the chill in your toes on a comforting hot water bottle. This is better. This is MUCH better.

8:39pm

Doing okay. A little edgy but okay. I think I got a little stressed about what Dr Hamilton was talking to me about earlier. Quiet day required tomorrow I think.

5th October 8:46am

Feeling a little paranoid (what's new?) this morning but generally okay. What am I paranoid about? The usual — that Pam, Nikki and Kim are talking about me and plotting against me behind my back. It's a horrible sensation/feeling/whatever and whilst I've learned to realise that it isn't real try telling my head that (or at least the part that needs convincing). I don't need a PRN right now. I can cope with this. And I WILL.

12:20pm

Lasted until now to take a PRN — not bad going when you consider how rotten I feel at the moment and how LOOPY my brain is going about Kim and Nikki and, to a lesser extent, Pam. I'm sure Kim and Nikki HATE me but I don't really want to do anything proactive about it right now. Maybe (definitely) I'm being a coward but I'm kind of hoping it'll just fade into the ether with the PRN.

2:15pm

You know, aside from the paranoia (which SUCKS) today has been all right. No really solid suicidal thoughts, no hallucinations, a good time out with Mum. So I can't complain. I guess.

I'm still feeling a bit edgy about the nurses on duty today but EVEN I realise that whilst they might be saying awful things about me they're NOT going to HARM ME and this is just paranoia spinning its web all around my brain. The problem is that my thoughts get caught in the web and the more they struggle the more enmeshed they become until they can't get free or move at all. All they can do is sit there helplessly until the HORRIBLE paranoia spider comes along to NAIL them. Again and again. Over and over. Again and again. And so on...

4:15pm

I feel like **SHIT**. No fancy adjectives or nouns. Just SHIT. I HATE THIS. And I refuse to feel like this for much longer. What's going through my head right now? Well, there's:

1) Kim and Nikki are talking about me behind my back.
2) All of the staff hate me.
3) Pam is writing awful things about me in my notes.
4) I am more trouble than I'm worth.
5) I am stressed to bits.
6) I hate myself for all of this.

7:52pm

Doing better after a chat with Pam and a PRN. Had a strange experience around 6pm. I went for a walk down to Costcutter's, saw a bus coming towards me along the main road and decided NOT to jump in front of it, took about 10 steps when ZOOM this black bird flies out of the hedge SO CLOSE TO MY FACE THAT IT BRUSHES MY CHEEK WITH ITS WINGS. Weird. Not God or fate. Just weird. And kind of life affirming too (in a non cheesy way).

Thankfully the paranoia has mostly backed off just leaving a residue of mild suspicion and uncomfortable — ness around people. Hopefully that will have gone by tomorrow and I'll be in sparkling form for my MDT.

10:01pm

KERRRIIIST! It just keeps on firing back like a paranoia boomerang! LEAVE ME ALONE!!!

6th October 7:56am

Right now I feel a bit crap and worried. I'm sure that Dr Hamilton is going to try and discharge me today whilst Dr Smith is away. I'm not going to write down what I think her plan is, suffice to say there IS one and it's against ME. This paranoia is like a bird that has flown, inadvertently, through an open window and is frantically flying around a room (my brain) desperately and randomly searching for the way out — the solution seems so obvious but getting there is SO difficult. I just wish I could put the thoughts in a box and BIN them. I guess the first step is finding the right box...

9:46am

Feeling a bit better but I can still feel the slow but definite drip of paranoia in the back regions of my head. It's okay and tolerable at the moment...that's all I can say really.

Anyway, I feel a little better about Dr Hamilton, which is cool.

10:50am

Too much going on in the Ward this morning so I'm going for a stroll in town. Feeling better though.

12:01pm

For some reason I got really nervous about handing this in! Mercifully Kim hadn't read it by the time I got back so I could retrieve it. Getting paranoid about being paranoid is NOT a good thing. No MDT today which is probably a good thing as my proposed double overnight would have coincided with his trip to London. His Mum is showing signs of kidney failure and her skin tone has changed — she is delirious too.

Mum just called and offered to take me out for coffee to Luss around 2:30pm so I'll see how I'm doing. Felt anxious after giving Kim the sweets I had got the staff — as though she'd think I was trying to blackmail her or something...or SOMETHING.

7:20pm

Took a PRN around 6:00pm because I believed that people were spying on me and talking about me — you know, the usual. I feel as though I am bouncing from PRN to PRN at the moment which kind of sucks. A lot. And I HOPE that Dr Smith knows what the solution is 'cos I don't.

8:08pm

Just reread this diary and it comes across as stupid, lame and pathetic. Hmmm. Me too, I guess.

7th October 8:40am

Tough morning. AND I ended up sounding like a 5 year old to Kim. Let's see if I can do better here: last night I had a really constructive chat with Dorothy about my paranoia and I felt as though we made some progress with methods of dealing with it.

However, this morning I felt the spiky glove of paranoia tightening its grip so I went for a walk and, on my return, the whole conspiracy theory thing kicked off when I discovered that Maxine (Student Nurse) was to be my allocated nurse for the day>student nurses get easy/discharge patients>they've given up on me>I have NO chance>everyone wants me dead>I HAVE NO CHANCE>AAAAAARRGGHH! Staff/Docs/family/friends are all against me.

I had a chat with Kim after breakfast which helped a bit but I STILL feel isolated and persecuted plus I didn't really believe the whole "Maxine has more time for you" line. I KNOW I am being unfair but I'm just scared that's all.

12:21pm

I think my overall concern here is that the staff will conclude that this plateau that I have reached is ME well. At least ME well enough to go home. But it's NOT. I wouldn't be able to cope at home for long like this. It would be HORRENDOUS. Really. And that whole idea SCARES THE SHIT OUT OF ME. The paranoia is still at too much of a severity and a frequency for me to cope with. Don't get me wrong, I DO want to go home...just not feeling like THIS. I'm still finding overnight stays a bit of a struggle, never mind the full Monty. But, if there is a conspiracy against me there's damn all I can do about it is there?

1:10pm

Feeling a bit better but I KNOW that my thoughts and feeling feel 100% spot on even if others contest them. I just KNOW.

5:01pm

Spoke to Dr Hamilton and then Dr Fallowfield about the thoughts I have been having. I didn't see the point in not being candid. I'm scared to bits 70% of the time and the other 30% isn't too shiny either. Dr Hamilton allayed my fears of a conspiracy by the staff/medics against me as did Dr Fallowfield who also helped me to understand WHY this is happening – the process at least. I THINK I believe them. But I'm not totally sure. I never really am about anything these days. I'm feeling okay at the moment and had a laugh with Alicia and Kim but even when I left them the suspicions about what they were saying and planning were growing...

8:57pm

Knackered. But my cheeseburger was mighty fine. So that was nice.

8th October 8:10am

I'm feeling okay this morning but (and you just KNEW there was a "but" coming) I am really tired and feeling a touch vulnerable. Hopefully that will wear off and everything will be cool. Working on distraction techniques so they should keep me busy,

9:40am

Feeling a bit suspicious of staff but I'm coping pretty well so far. Going to get 10:ooam meds and head into town for a saunter.

10:51am

Nervous of talking on my phone as I AM SURE people are spying on me and listening in on my conversations. I'm worried about staff in general, especially talking to them. JUST LEAVE ME ALONE!!!

12:20pm
AAAAARRRGGGH! I'm SO TIRED of feeling suspicious and afraid!!!

1:42pm
I was given a PRN about an hour ago and I'm feeling much better. I can actually relax on my bed and doze without worry which is GREAT! Y'know what? Paranoia is scary, horrible and foul but it is also frustrating and limiting. Generally though not always, I REALISE I am paranoid but that does damn all to make it GO AWAY. THAT'S when I want to start SCREAMING. I feel hemmed in, trapped and stuck between a rock and a hard place. It's ROTTEN.

9th October 2:55pm
I've had a good day so far. The trip to Lomond Shores with Kathleen went well although I'm impatient and I want to get better in every way a lot FASTER. I think that's mainly because I'm getting patches of feeling like ME now which is good...for me at least!

Why is it that whilst the bad thoughts recede they NEVER TOTALLY go away? They grumble away in the background and are uneasy companions in my head. I just want to get shot of them completely. Mind you, at least there's no sign of paranoia today, at least not much — a little on the Ward and some at Lomond Shores but nothing I couldn't handle.

7:16pm
I spoke too soon. BAD thoughts and confusion fill my head and leer at me. I can't even get my head around packing my case for

tomorrow's pass — distraction technique no.215/f — so I've just chucked a bunch of clothes in and hoped for the best. The night staff have come on shift and already I'm quite nervous of them. Actually make that "quite scared". Why? Because I think they are thinking and plotting ways of "accidentally" harming me. I HATE THIS. I know what will happen: I'll face them, they'll deny it. AAAARRGGH! I KNOW this is paranoia.

Still feels like SHIT though.

8:37pm

Feeling a lot better. PRN has worked and I had a cheeseburger as a very effective distraction technique. I'm not kidding about the burger. There are so many valuable stages to getting a cheeseburger or, for that matter, ANY takeaway in a psychiatric Ward. For example, first of all you have to go to the staff and ask for a menu, then you decide what you want and see if you can afford it, then you phone the order, you then wait for the delivery car, if you're allowed you then go downstairs to let him in and finally you eat your takeaway (clearing up any mess you might have made afterwards eg washing dishes).

My head now feels more at ease with itself — as though there is less of a conflict going on internally. It was the right move, I think, to get the PRN and face the staff early on rather than just let it build. This seems to have nipped it in the bud earlier rather than later.

10th October 10:33am

Slept well and cuddled Mitch all night. He was wandering around in a bit of a daze this morning when the district nurse called in to update him on how things are with his Mum. The news, as we knew, isn't good — she is very frail now and fading fast. I'm doing my very best to be strong for Mitch right now but I can't be physically with him all the time. I've told him that I'll get the bus back to the Ward on my own so that he can stay and spend some time with his Mum. Me? I feel as though I am holding things together JUST BARELY but, as that's all I've got on offer just now I guess it has to be good enough.

12th October 11:51am

I am two people. I am safe. I am in grave danger. I am here. I am gone. I know a way out of this. I am hopelessly lost. I am clued up. I don't know what the Hell is going on. I am lurching between the two and the nausea I am feeling is a welcome respite from this confusion.

I want to go for a walk but I JUST DON'T KNOW. (Jesus, please make SOMETHING straightforward.) I WANT OFF THE WARD. Ultimately I have to take responsibility for my life. I just don't know how responsible I feel right now. Or what I feel capable of. I want shortbread. I'm not hungry. I am stable. I am all over the place.

1:49pm

I need to go and buy some coke (cos I'm about to run out) but I don't know how I feel about being a "big girl" and coping with going off the Ward. Mum just called to say they're off to see Megan, my other brother's newly born second daughter, so that's nice and I sent my best wishes.

4:41pm

Ever WANTED to do something but been scared of it at the same time? I guess bungee jumping, sky diving or getting a tattoo all fall into these categories but the reward — the adrenalin rush — is all too apparent whereas killing yourself offers nothing. But maybe that's the point. The "nothing" it offers is everything in contrast to the NIGHTMARE that is going on in your head.

I have spent today thinking long and hard about this. My conclusion? If I was alone in the World or in the perfect isolated vacuum I would do it simply because I couldn't STAND being on my own with this SHIT. But I'm NOT. I'm lucky enough to have Mitch, my family and my friends. And they seem to want me to stick around. Besides the "noise" has backed off a bit so that makes life easier — a lot easier in fact. I can actually think and act rationally as opposed to the messed up gnarly chaos that I live with sometimes. I think I'm learning to live more comfortably in my skin again. About time!

13th October 7:04pm

Have felt pretty good today (so far) apart from a nervy MDT and a bit of derealisation shortly afterwards. However, I was able to keep resolutely PRN — less. I'm still a bit confused as to why this is the greater good but my grasp of the conversation is a little tainted at the moment so I'm not quite sure of all the reasoning. I KNOW that when I ask for them my plea is genuine — it is not in my interest to take medication that I do not require, or that will not benefit me and...and I get scared about how I feel and want it sorted QUICKLY. PRNs help. But when

I'm living from PRN to PRN that situation is not satisfactory for either me or anyone involved in my care. So what of my baseline anti psychotic? Does the PRN use indicate it is not effective. I'm NO pharmacist but "Hello?" the indicators are there surely? Or maybe I just need to get my shit together better and try harder without PRNs? Maybe I'll wake up one day and everything will be just fine. Maybe.

Passes: Tues/Wed
         Fri/Sat/Sun

9:39pm

Today HAS been a good day but one thing has been baffling me: exactly WHAT is it about Michel that makes me love him so much? His wicked sense of humour? Probably. The fact that he is the smartest man I know by A MILE yet remains blissfully lacking in arrogance. And that he has the kindest heart that I have ever seen. Definitely. Yeah, today has been okay. Heh, heh.

14th October 7:52am

If I could put into words how I feel right now I'd probably make a FORTUNE 'cos I'm sure I'm LOADS of people go through this — I'm not that special. I feel the way a car feels when it stalls, the way your brain knows that split second faster than your leg that your leg has been broken in an accident, the way you KNOW when someone is playing out of tune in an orchestra even though you can't sing a note in key to save your life. I feel all of this and more. Yes, I thought about killing myself on my walk this morning but, equally, I also thought A LOT about why I

shouldn't. The shouldn'ts now far outweigh the shoulds (obviously).
Will this always be the case. Honestly? I don't know.

I think part of my problem is that I don't believe in myself. Maybe
I need to start to.

2:01pm
Feeling okay – a bit paranoid about Kim – but hey, what's new?
As you can tell the paranoia is at a level that I'm coping with so
generally I'm fine.

3:35pm
Waiting for Dr Fallowfield...and trying to keep a lid on the awful
thoughts that I'm having. I feel like I'm a TERRIBLE person and
that everyone HATES me. I'm nervous and worried. But I think
I can handle this. Maybe. I'll talk to Dr Fallowfield.

Just bumped into Kim who smiled at me as did Dr Hamilton and
Una. Stupid I know but little reassurances impact and make me
feel better. It pisses me off as to how sensitive and vulnerable
my mood/paranoia state is. GRRRRRR!!!

15th October 4:50pm
Everything in Michel's house REEKS of death. Diamorphine lies
on his Mum's desk. The air doesn't seem to move. It makes me
feel sick. It really does. Which is why I was the coward who bailed
and came back to the Ward rather than stay and endure the
when? When? When? With Mitch. I can't hack this. Part of me
is trying to get better. Part of me is trying to be strong, stronger,
strongest for someone else.

At times I feel like I'm drowning.
It's not a good feeling.

16th October 8:59am

I feel like my skin is coated in black, oily cling film this morning that is choking my pores and making breathing difficult. I must have sat for about 20 mins in reception giving it "Should I/Shouldn't I?". The answer might have been in doubt but the question never was. I think the fact that I can still pose myself such questions, and so seriously as well, scares the shit out of me. I'm not messing around here — this is the crap that goes around and around inside my head at times and it's HORRENDOUS. But I'M STILL HERE.

Did I think I would get to this stage? Of course not! At least not for a LONG time. But I have. And if I were to spend the rest of my life saying "thank you" it still wouldn't be even CLOSE enough to adequately thank those who have helped me.

1:50pm

Okay. So things were pretty good. My lunch out with Kathleen was successful and I felt positive and confident about things. And then? And then I come back from a walk and Katy looks at me funny, as does Kathleen and suddenly I feel as though I am the leper of the Ward and everyone hates me. I'm stressed out and my head is all over the place. GODDAMNIT.

I'm supposed to go through this whole discharge plan with Katy today but I'm nervous. More than that I'm nervous of being nervous so I hope we get it sorted today.

2:28pm

Feeling better again. Had a bit of banter with Pam and Kathleen about how they were to quit analysing each other. Why? BECAUSE IT FRIES THEIR BRAINS!!!

5:46pm

I'm a little (LOT) concerned that if I'm not supposed to be taking so many PRNs (fair enough) why am I STILL experiencing episodes like this morning? I KNOW I got through it without one but I felt like shit and it went on longer because of that. How do I know I have reached a satisfactory level of recovery to go home and, if I don't know, how will the staff and doctors gauge it??? Okay, I reckon I WILL figure when the time is right but this recovery business isn't the smoothest of roads so it is in my interest that EVERYONE (including me) knows where I'm headed and how to get there. This whole process needs to be done GRADUALLY because I'm SCARED and it needs to be done right if it is to achieve the ultimate goal. You know what I mean — living a positive, constructive happy and worthwhile life in the presence/absence of symptoms. THAT is what I want...preferably in the ABSENCE of symptoms, or else managed successfully.

Is that realistic or just bare faced greed?

17th October 8:05am

Woke up in a GOOD mood this morning after going to sleep following an amusing discussion with Nurse Lydia mainly over the correct spelling of the delightful term boak/boke — the pronunciation was NEVER in question! B...O...A...K!!! Aaah, the things we learn in life!

6:45 pm

Slept all afternoon after a brief visit to Michel's Mums's and a coffee in town. All that and a trip to the Supermarket fried my brain a bit and so I took a PRN and went to bed for a bit for a bit of recuperation time.

10:46pm

On one hand today went well — no disasters. On the other hand it strikes me how much more DIFFICULT I find everything than I used to: choosing yoghurt in the Supermarket, talking to people in the street, deciding how much money to spend on something etc. I love Mitch to pieces but when he wanted me to choose where to go for a coffee in town I really floundered. We've just finished talking about it and I figure I need three things to help me get my head together out of the Ward: 1. less pressure 2. reassurance 3. a little responsible guidance until I find my feet.

I'm not some kid by any means but I've just spent 7 months away from society and that's going to mess up anyone's head.

18th October 10:11am

Somebody turned off the gravity at around 1:00am last night 'cos all Hell broke loose and everything, although in many ways expected, still managed to shock, harass and upset. I've never seen a dead person before and I think it was the stillness of the room and THAT smell which bothered me most. Poor Mitch. He played a blinder in the "holding it together stakes" but he was pale and a bit shaky. I held his hand and willed him good thoughts. So, we took a cab to the house, met with the Marie Curie nurse, waited for the on call GP, and then waited for the undertaker, each meeting presenting fresh challenges and methodical heartache. Neither Mitch nor I slept much once we got back home so we are going to just cuddle up and spend today in bed.

19th October 12:15pm

Didn't sleep too well and I'm knackered from the last few days but, in retrospect, I think it was important for Mitch's and my relationship that I was there for him. Tough though. And I CAN'T GET his Mum's dead face out of my head.

Just back at the Ward and I can stop coping now. Putting on a brave face all the time sucks a bit and I need to relax and come to terms with how I feel about the last few days. But I also realise that I am NOT the most important person in this horrible situation and I need to look out for Mitch who is. How do I feel? Kind of sick, tired and a bit all over the place emotionally. Nothing unusual really, given the circumstances.

4:14pm

Got to sort out a pass for the funeral and put in a request for pass meds etc. Feeling pretty depressed right now. I don't really understand this much I mean, I realise that the death of anyone is a shock but I felt that, for reasons of self protection, I had said "goodbye" several weeks ago and had moved on so that I could be strong for Mitch. So much for that plan.

I DON'T NEED BEREAVEMENT COUNSELLING (though I think it's a good idea for Mitch). I just need to get through this by talking it through with staff (humour allowed) and by helping organise the cremation with Mitch. I need to feel like I'm doing the right thing by Mitch as far as this whole thing goes. Oh yeah...I'M KNACKERED.

20th October 8:17am

Last night was awful. Paranoia crawled all over me in increasing waves and just when I thought I had it beat (or at least under control) BOOM! A fresh new torrent would rise up and overwhelm me. Fuck. I suppose it could be measured by my phone call pattern 1. could take calls in the 4 bedded dorm>2. could only take calls in the unlocked 4 bedded bathroom>3. door locked>4. could only take calls in corridor bathroom, door locked/whispering. The reason for all of this was that I was growing increasingly SURE that my calls were being listened to and monitered. Two things happened as a consequence: A) I thought I was going to have to speak in code or else my AMAZINGLY uninteresting phone calls were going to be dissected and pawed over. B) I handed my phone in to the office to get it out of my face and out of my head. Dumb, I know but it worked.

The reason for all this bollocks? Grief fucking with me. I'm really trying SO HARD to keep Mitch's head on straight that I think that mine wobbled a bit last night. Plus it's hard to come up with positive distraction techniques when you're knackered but not yet ready to go to sleep.

This morning I feel better and more in control. I've got my phone back and I feel okay about it. I'll call Mitch at 9:00am and see how he's doing.

11:55am

Had a pretty good morning and managed to get everything I was to organise organised for the service on Wed.

4:47pm

GOOD MDT. Sat there shaking like the proverbial for ¾ of it but managed to stutter and stammer my way vaguely coherently through it. Dr Smith and I chatted casually about aspects of death before broaching the topic of cremations and interments. Nah, the MDT WAS a good one. Really. Dr Smith is happy that my mood is improved but is a tad concerned about my lithium level so blood test tomorrow to check things out. Also...meeting with Dr Hamilton tomorrow to chat about DISCHARGE PLANS! All systems GGGGGGGOOOOOOO!!!!!!

21st October...

22nd October 9:45pm

Why is it that on days when the weather is supposed to be AMAZING (birthdays, holidays etc) it LASHES down and yet on crap days when the weather is supposed to match your mood it turns up all shiny and sunny???

The service was small and lovely and I was SO PROUD of Mitch and the touching eulogy that he delivered. He is a fantastic guy and he's been holding it together really well (maybe a little TOO well – I worry about him). After the cremation we all headed to the Buffet Shop for some breakfast where I made the effort to be assertive and put myself in charge of placing our orders.

Small steps. After breakfast we went up to my Mum's where I unfortunately slept all afternoon and generally felt rubbish until about 6:30pm when we had dinner. Mitch and I headed to bed early and I gave him loads of hugs. He's doing okay and I'm all right.

I had one episode of paranoia at breakfast today when I was sure everyone was staring at me and talking about me. But I got through it. Which was cool. I just convinced myself that I'm REALLY not that interesting and try and immerse myself in a conversation with someone near to me. What do you know? It worked.

23rd October 1:16pm

Woke up this morning feeling pretty crap and edgy and as the morning progressed so did the crapness, misery and terrifying bad thoughts. I was pretty agitated in the house and figured that as I was PRN – less it would be best for me to come back early to the Ward. I feel like shit at the moment AND my stomach's acting up.

Haven't asked for a PRN yet because I feel scared of the staff and their questions.

4:36pm

Feeling MUCH better mentally. Sorted out my care plan with Katy which all looks pretty fine. I'm kind of torn though – part of me wants to go home NOW for good, whereas part of me says "No, do this right and take your time". What to do, what to do, what to do?!! I think I'll pick the sensible option and stay put for now 'cos I've been here before in previous admissions and I REALLY want to avoid that revolving door.

7:10pm

I'm finding it remarkable as to how intimidated and nervous I'm feeling when I'm talking to/with staff. It sucks and I hate it. It makes me shake all the more. GRRRR! I am 35 years old and supposed to be an adult. Yeah right!

24th October 8:39am

Still a bit shaky but at least I'm not twitching. Other than that I'm okay. I need to speak to Kathleen about how my social phobia challenge is progressing what with various occasions coming up as Xmas approaches. Feel pretty damn anxious today and I have NO IDEA why.

1:42pm

Feeling good — just been for a walk in the pissing rain and managed not to drown! Bumped into a local GP who I know which was both unexpected and lovely. I coped with the meeting with less nerves and more control than I expected which was cool. I actually managed eye contact and was able to make sense. Shaky though.

8:04pm

I had a great afternoon but now? Now paranoia haunts me and I feel nervous, suspicious and vulnerable and I HATE IT. I am in a total agony of deciding whether I should approach staff or hide in my room. Shit. AND I've got that electric shock feeling on my arms which isn't good. This has been building up since 5:00pm ish and I DON'T KNOW WHY!

25th October 7:55am

Paranoia sucks. Nervous as Hell of Katy and Gary and wary of whoever else approaches my room.

8:05am

Breakfast was horrible. I felt like someone was jabbing pins into me all over my body and I was certain that the staff were/are talking about me and taking the piss. Just had a PRN so hopefully things should improve. They've got to be better than last night when I was SURE that everything that the staff said was a "test" e.g. "How are you?"> TEST "Any shakes"> TEST. I'm still not sure what was going on in my head there but the consequence was avoiding staff as much as possible and not engaging with them. I was just scared. That's all.

5:45pm

IT NEVER RAINS BUT IT POURS...

26th October

Feel a bit out of it and confused this morning. Nothing seems real. Derealisation I think, which sucks. I'm really missing Mitch — he's away on business — I even wore his shoes to the hairdressers so that he could, in a way, keep me company while I was there.

5:45pm

Had a lovely visit from my friend Lisa and her family but pretty tired now. Back to the Ward, dyed hair, had a cup of coffee and a small chat with Dorothy. Now lying on bed just thinking.........I can't compromise on what I want to feel and this is NOT HOW

I WANT TO FEEL. I can't afford to feel like I really want to be dead when I am alone at home and, let's face it folks, that day WILL happen. Maybe I'm being melodramatic but I'm just a bit/lot scared that's all. Of course none of us can be certain about our futures I fully realise that. I just want everyone (and ME) to be able to feel comfortable that I will manage. THIS IS NOT COMING OUT RIGHT!!! I feel really shaky, edgy and unhappy just now and I don't know what to do about it. I feel like my body has been turned inside out and all my skin is raw, bleeding and being attacked by EVERYTHING. STOP. JUST FUCKING STOP. PLEASE!

I can't even open the MAIL at the moment without getting stressed out to the max never mind actually coping with bills etc. How on earth am I going to organise myself when I go home? I WANT to be independent and I don't like this person that I have turned into – all needy and pathetic. I'm better, SO MUCH BETTER – I can see that, so where does all this TERROR come from?

9:14pm
Feeling calmer. I'll be okay. Even made up a crap joke: What do you call a turkey on prozac? A Perkey!!!

28th October 1:02pm
Spoke to Katy about my upcoming trip to London for the interment of his Mum's ashes, and found that really hard and anxiety provoking. She's freaking me out today and it's doing my HEAD IN....actually so's Kim (what a shock!) so it's nothing personal!

4:44pm

Dr Fallowfield and I talked about the paranoia and anxiety that might arise in London and ways of combating them. We also spoke about me projecting thoughts, feelings and expectations onto other people and reflecting them back (if you get my drift). He then got all the paranoid hairs on the back of my neck to stand on end by moving his chair back while we were speaking> he's not interested>I'm boring and crap. Champion. There are so many times when I think I have this beat then BAM!!!! It jumps all over me. I've had the shakes ever since.

8:03pm

STILL feeling edgy and paranoid despite a PRN/a cheeseburger with extra relish and salad and a packet of bacon fries. Ah bollocks. I'm just going to lie low and HOPEFULLY this HORRIBLE feeling that everyone HATES me and that I have done something terribly wrong will get lost.

I think things are a bit difficult right now NOT because I am going backwards — quite the opposite in fact — but because I am at this transitionary stage of passes home/time on the Ward etc and it's all a bit unsettling, NECESSARY, but unsettling. However I would rather do it this way than rush things too much and end up back here in 3 months time. The big picture is that everything is going well it's just that I get caught up in the details sometimes and get myself in a right mess.

29th October 1:19pm

Was hurtled to Clydebank by my Mum and we had a pretty good time talking, window shopping and eventually finding O J a birthday present which is a....wait for it....cool as anything black leather coat. It's double breasted and looks awesome. So that's him sorted from me and Mitch, then.

Stopped off at McDonald's on the way back – rude not to – and talked to Mum a LITTLE bit about the battle I had had with suicidal thoughts and plans during my time on the Ward. It just felt like the right moment and so, sitting in McDonald's car park I opened up a touch about what had been parading noisily around my head and she, in turn, spoke about how desperately worried they had all been about my physical state. I think both of us learned a bit about either end of the spectrum of my illness. Scary stuff but (hopefully) in the past.

Oddly, I was never really THAT worried about the physical side. Sure, I was puking my head off and feeling AWFUL but I was SO MUCH MORE distracted with what was going on in my head that everything else was secondary and if I died? So be it, for all I care. It was a LOUSY place to be to be honest and I never intend to return there again.

2:05pm
Got the shakes.

4:20pm
Little paranoia daggers are starting to jab at me again which is making it awkward to be around staff. I WILL approach them before the stabbing gets too persistent and keeps me away for good.

November

3rd November 8:55am

Feeling REALLY anxious this morning. Not sure why. Actually that's a lie and a BIG FAT BLACK ONE at that. I'd ask Dorothy for a chat or even a PRN but hey, I'm TOO ANXIOUS. AAAAAAAAAAARRRGH!!!!!

I'm not sure how I'm going to cope with what's ahead of me in my life but 2 things are sure: 1. I HAVE to 2. I WANT to which, let's face it, are BIG improvements on how things were even a couple of months ago. Even I can see that. Flipping heck.

Had a HUGE chat with Kim last night about how I feel as though I don't belong anywhere – I'm too well for the Ward/not well enough to cope 24/7 at home – I realise I have to follow a proper discharge plan or else I'll end up back in here pretty damn soon which would NOT be fun and laughter, so they'll be no rash decisions from me. I think the plan Dr Hamilton laid out is the right one and is the one I'll follow. Even answering the phone or opening a letter at home freaks me out right now so I think "graduated exposure" are the words I'm searching for.

8:30pm

Paranoia's crap. But at least it's a damn sight milder than it used to be. Right now part of me believes that one of my roommates is only pretending to be asleep and is actually spying on me. The rest of me? The rest of me thinks that's RUBBISH. But it is still banging resolutely around my head and pissing me off royally.

Other than that today had been okay. I've found that in order to keep and cope with a secret I've had to disclose it. Which kind of makes sense — to me at least. And I've had to confront my anxiety issues — particularly those surrounding the secret — I'm hoping that with the help of Dorothy and Kathleen I can overcome them.

The BIGGEST problem I have (not right now, but maybe sometime...) is how the fuck do I get off this horrific travelator that I seem to be superglued to. I have this awful fixed idea about where it ends up. And NOTHING I seem to do helps. EVERYTHING feels bigger than me and I am powerless to change things. I realise that I have huge choices to face and I'm REALLY hoping I can do this right. I guess I just HAVE to. Of course I realise that I am being a miserable, nihilistic sod here but I can't apologise because my mind's eye is a scary place to be. I'm not talking about tomorrow, next month or even next year. Honestly I have NO idea — maybe HOPEFULLY, NEVER. So far? I am still here.

I would SO MUCH like for these thoughts to GO AWAY and leave me feeling more secure about things, especially for when I go home.

4th November 2:21pm

Haven't done much today because I'm feeling pretty horrible physically — totally knackered and poorly — so I've just slept all day (barring a trip to the canteen to get some soup). I've got my period too which probably isn't helping. Mentally I'm doing okay though so that's cool.

3:57pm

Feeling worse — sick, shaky and tired. Moan, moan, moan.

Awaiting LFTs.

6th November 2:36pm

LFTs fine on Tuesday. Still feeling a bit shaky and tired. Ah well. LOTS GOING ON (at the moment anyway) but I think it's time I realised my limitations and recognised that I have been through the wringer (just a teensy bit) this year. As such I think that in deference to self preservation I should take things easy and not leap head first into the deep end with no arm bands to keep me afloat. Plus, as it was rightly pointed out to me there is (I hope) a lot more to me than bipolar and perhaps I should be focusing on those aspect for the moment.

9th November 10:00am

Cuddled up to Mitch and feeling safe, relaxed and secure. HOME. At least, ONE aspect. As are bills, emails, money, housework, stress etc. AM I READY???

2:00pm

Anxiety and paranoia scrape their claws down my bones, clattering and rattling my innards like rigid, wind filled sails in an Autumn storm. I WANT TO GO HOME. But "I want to go home" is a bit like a tired elastoplast covering "Am I ready?" and "Could I cope?". Of these things I have to be as certain as I can because I DON'T WANT TO RETURN.

I think the anxiety I am experiencing is definitely worse on the Ward but is PRIMARILY aggravated by the fact that I feel unsettled at home AND on the Ward — neither feels like a place I belong to at the moment. The paranoia is LOVING this and, if I'm honest, it's freaking me out.

So, I've given myself 2 WEEKS to get it together, spending the vast majority of my time at home with Mitch (but I know the Ward is there in the background should I need it) and then? Then hopefully I can begin to live again and put this 7½ month stutter behind me. Right now I feel 4 things: 1. Sick 2. Realistically positive and enthusiastic about the future for the first time in AGES 3. ANXIOUS 4. Nervous of Lydia (whom I will continue to avoid). However the bad stuff isn't NEARLY as bad as it used to be (although the anxiety is a BITCH) and I can hack it all much better than I used to.

11th November 10:54am

Shaky as anything but NOT feeling anxious. What's that all about???

Good family celebration last night for Ollie's 30th — Chinese take away — always goes down well (especially when the take away is giving away FREEBIES!!!). Mitch and I sat down to watch "Spooks" afterwards and as such spent most of the following hour yelling "Bollocks!" at the TV. (The TV didn't bat an eyelid). How this relates to my mental state I am unsure but I certainly feel okay.

Mum, Mitch and Ollie off to Stirling Uni this morning to chat about mental health to students. I decided it would be wiser for me NOT to go as the phrases "Leaping into deep water" and "Without a life jacket" spring to mind when I think of speaking to any number of people (eg 1) at the moment.

Speaking of which...chatted to Alicia for a bit around 9:00 ish which was fine but got difficult when others joined the conversation and the numbers went up.

16th November 8:46pm

Today has been good, barring a snotty cold, the odd minor burst of paranoia and anxiety (saying goodbye to people ALWAYS sucks.) The question I need to deal with is "Are these symptoms something I'm prepared to put up with?" Obviously I'd like them to sod right off but is that ever really going to happen? God, I hope so. ALL of the symptoms I present with are SO limiting in that they scare the pants off me and cause me to hide and withdraw, socially at least. I get suspicious of everyone at times BUT those times are a LOT less and I'm doing well (I think). The anxiety (and the shakes) are ROTTEN but I am determined to beat them — I just need some time and support, I guess (Jesus, could I SOUND more pathetic?)

I NEED to go home. That is not the question. "When" is. Because I've got to do this right as I have ABSOLUTELY no intentions of ending up in any "revolving door" that anyone cares to speak of. So. No messing. I don't want to stay too long but equally I don't want to go too soon. And this is NO game. No way.

19th November 9:05am

FINALLY. *And believe me, there were* PLENTY *of times when I never thought it would happen, I'm getting discharged tomorrow. Of course this road I'm walking down hasn't suddenly ended (although now I'm striding purposely as opposed to crawling on my hands and knees) and I* KNOW *there will be bumps and troughs along the way but* FUCK *I've come a long way. Further than I ever imagined was possible.*

From April 1st through to whenever the Hell it was that I was back on a therapeutic level of medication I SCREAMED *with every ounce of my being that I* NEEDED HELP *right form the early onset of my psychosis in the acute medical Ward through to my 6 ½ months residency in Christie Ward where that scream echoed, reverberated and, at times, overwhelmed me.*

So, I KNEW *I needed help but without medication I was pretty damn certain I was fucked — I was either going to kill myself or, in my paranoid world, someone else was. Neither happened. What* DID *happen during those 7½ months is that I lost myself several times over and at times I honestly believed there was no way back from the horrific places I found myself in. How do you get through something like that?* You TRY REALLY HARD NOT TO QUIT *but when you* DO *quit (and you do) you turn to those around you and place everything about yourself in their hands. You have to or it's game over.*

What I'm trying to express here is just how GOBSMACKINGLY *important Christie Ward and its nursing staff are. They saved my life. It doesn't come any more black or white than that.*

These 7 ½ months have been the HARDEST THING that I have EVER done and they held my hand, talked to me, took away my fucking shoelaces, listened, counselled me, offered coping techniques, helped me integrate, made me smile when I never thought I would again and, more than anything, helped me believe that mine was a life worth living even though before I had thought all was lost. They gave me 6 words:

I AM GOING TO MAKE IT

........I just need to keep believing that.

THE END

Epilogue

One year on....

On the 17th April 2009, Michel and I were married in St Andrews, Fife (where I went to University). It was a beautiful service – just Michel, myself, two witnesses and a Registrar present and, without a shadow of a doubt, the happiest day of my life.

There were many times over the past year when I was unsure – maybe more than unsure – that I would make it to our wedding. Viral Hepatitis A was a thief who had stolen my barricades which had been carefully constructed to keep out psychosis. Imagine the frustration that I felt at medication time when I could SEE the medication I used to take on the "drug trolley" about one and a half metres from me and yet I WAS FORBIDDEN from taking it. I resented the other patients as they easily swallowed down pills which offered sanity and sleep.

You might have noticed that I haven't mentioned that many of the other patients in this book – that's for privacy reasons but there is one story I would like to recount. I had been on the Ward for about three weeks and had hardly said a word to anyone (apparently my nickname was "Growler" amongst the other patients!). I was sitting curled up on a seat in reception when one of the male patients came in through the main door carrying two cups of coffee, some sugar and some portions of milk. "There you go." He said as he placed a coffee in front of me "You look like you could do with this." Then without waiting for me to stir or utter any words he turned on his heel and headed down the corridor. Sometimes kindness takes your breath away.

I've been back to the Ward twice since I was discharged – once to visit Katy and once to pick up some documents that I had left behind. How did I find it? Difficult. The minute I stepped through the main door ghosts of memories past swamped me and I began to shake uncontrollably. It's frustrating because I really wanted the staff to see that I'm doing okay and coping in the community. This will come, I'm sure. One thing I hope I've made clear in this book is that when you are discharged from an acute psychiatric Ward you are not suddenly "better", you are merely part of the way on the road to recovery and there is still an awful lot of work to be done in the community to keep you well (or at least well enough to stay out of hospital).

I like to think I am fairly articulate on the written page but it wasn't until last year and my stay in Christie that I really understood the meanings of the words empathy, care, insight, observation and professionalism. The nurses and auxiliaries taught me well.

Finally, there is something lacking in medical Wards in hospitals around our country…an understanding of mental illness and psychiatry. I am NOT expecting medical nurses to be expert in psychiatry but when you take into consideration that there are 1 in 4 people suffering from a mental illness at any time and that each dorm in a Ward has 4 beds what does that tell you? Surely some proficiency would be of benefit to everyone. I recall suffering a stream of hallucinations and I was greeted with a "Sorry, we don't do psychiatry" when I was on the acute medical Ward. Even having a psychiatric nurse covering the medical Ward would be a start so that they could be beeped if there was a problem. Something must be done to break down the divide and misunderstandings between medical nurses and psychiatric ones.

The community team that works with me now is fantastic and it's always good to know that the CRISIS (out of hours) team and Breathing Space are there at the end of a phone line should I need them. But most of all I find it incredibly exciting to be able to think and plan for the future – a future that not so long ago I thought that I had lost forever.

The Naked Bird Watcher

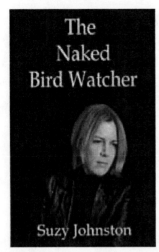

by Suzy Johnston,
ISBN 0954809203

In an engaging, informative and often amusing autobiography, what continually shines through is the author's consistently positive outlook and her refusal to be ashamed of losing what she describes as 'the battle of percentages' in developing manic depression. In this candid and honest description of one person's experience of living a full and varied life whilst coping with a serious mental health problem, the author gives a vivid but lucid insight into the torment that is mental distress, while highlighting the importance of good psychiatric treatment, support and self management as the vital aids to recovery which will be of immense value, help and reassurance to many.

The Snow Globe Journals
by Suzy Johnston,
ISBN 9780954809225

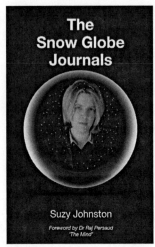

The Snow Globe Journals

Suzy Johnston

Foreword by Dr Raj Persaud
'The Mind'

Suzy Johnston broke new ground in personal account of recovery from mental illness in her outstanding autobiography The Naked Bird Watcher. Building on issues raised in that first book, The Snow Globe Journals charts first-hand the daily experience and challenges facing anyone with a long-term mental conditon - from psychosis, feelings of suicide, paranoia and the compulsion to self-harm through to being admitted to and living in a psychiatric ward and the staging posts in the long road to recovery.

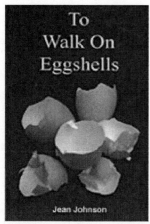

To Walk on Eggshells
by Jean Johnston,
ISBN 0954809211

Facing the challenge of looking after mental illness is frightening and isolating. I hope this account of my experiences and how I felt, along with what I learnt, will help to alleviate the loneliness of their situation as they face the challenge of being 'The Carers' of mental illness with the book perhaps offering some reassurance

LaVergne, TN USA
29 July 2010
191396LV00001B/76/P